A
MARIHUANA
DICTIONARY

A
MARIHUANA
DICTIONARY

Words, Terms, Events,
and Persons Relating to Cannabis

ERNEST L. ABEL

GREENWOOD PRESS
Westport, Connecticut • London, England

Library of Congress Cataloging in Publication Data

Abel, Ernest L., 1943-
    A marihuana dictionary.

    Bibliography: p.
    Includes index.
    1. Marihuana—dictionaries.   I. Title.
HV5822.M3A2   306'.1   81-13427
ISBN 0-313-23252-0 (lib. bdg.)   AACR2

Library of Congress Catalog Card Number 81-13427
ISBN: 0-313-23252-0

First published in 1982

Greenwood Press
A division of Congressional Information Service, Inc.
88 Post Road West, Westport, Connecticut 06881

Printed in the United States of America

10 9 8 7 6 5 4 3 2 1

CONTENTS

ACKNOWLEDGMENTS

Appreciation is extended to the many people who provided lists of terms. A special expression of appreciation is extended to Dr. Michael Aldrich, curator of the Fitzhugh Ludlow Library, for providing me with many sources that would otherwise have been difficult, if not impossible, to obtain; to Renee Bush, who proofread several versions of the manuscript and suggested many improvements; and to Dianne Augustino, librarian of the Research Institute on Alcoholism, who, as always, was very helpful in tracking down source material.

INTRODUCTION

Marihuana came of age in the United States in the 1960s.

Not that it was any new discovery. Marihuana, hashish, charas, kif, pot, grass, or whatever it was called had been around for thousands of years before it came to America.

Marihuana was introduced to Americans as a drug at the turn of the century, concealed in the little *mota* bags Mexican workers carried with them across the border. Before that, marihuana was called "hemp," and it was no stranger to the United States.

The hemp plant, *Cannabis sativa*, was brought to the New World by the early colonists, and both George Washington and Thomas Jefferson were hemp farmers. In those days, hardly a household in America didn't own something made of its tough, durable fibers. In some colonies hemp was so highly valued it was even accepted in place of money!

But for some unknown reason, Americans didn't think of chewing or smoking the leaves of the hemp plant until quite recently.

By the 1920s, marihuana had spread from the Mexican to the black communities of the South, and when Mexican and black workers migrated north in search of jobs, so did marihuana. By the 1930s, all the big cities had their marihuana "dealers" and buyers.

Worried that the drug might incite violence and sexual deviance, lawmakers around the country passed laws making it illegal. In 1937 Congress passed the Marihuana Tax Act, and marihuana went underground. Use of marihuana became a felony offense. In many states, conviction carried a long prison sentence; in some, a convicted marihuana user could be sentenced to death.

By the 1960s, however, white middle-class college students began using marihuana, and the lawmakers were faced with a personal predicament: Enforce the law and put their own sons and daughters in jail or change the law. By the 1970s, the laws against marihuana began to change. Marihuana still remained illegal. Now it was just less illegal.

Because of the fear of discovery and the consequences of such discovery, marihuana users had to find ways and means of keeping their drug usage secret. A key element in this clandestine effort was the development and refining of a special language—a lingo—by which users could communicate with one another and identify who was a user and who was not.

Lingos or argots, as students of language call them, have always been around. Every group has one. Doctors, lawyers, athletes, railway workers, musicians, and so on, all develop, refine, and perpetuate their own language within the general language. These lingos are passwords. They say "I belong."

Lingos are not developed to hide behind. Instead, they evolve as a way of fostering group solidarity. Those who use a particular lingo derive pleasure from it. They take pride in using it. They judge others by their knowledge of it. A lingo promotes camaraderie and cohesiveness because it reflects and embodies the thinking and life-styles—the attitudes, values, habits, concerns, fears, aspirations, and activities—of the group.

Like all slang, however, marihuana lingo is constantly changing. As soon as various terms become widely known to and used by the public, they are dropped and are replaced by new terms. Certain terms also tend to be regional. The same term may even have a different meaning in different parts of the country. But even with the ephemeral quality of much of the lingo, there always seems to be a core of terms that is perpetuated through generations as if it were a cultural heirloom. This colorful, cryptic heirloom is the main subject matter of this marihuana dictionary.

Marihuana lingo seems to intrigue both scholars and the general public. Scholars are fascinated by this language within a language because it offers new insights into America's drug culture. The general public seems just as fascinated by the colorful language, as witnessed by the many pop songs, movies, magazines, and books that contain marihuana jargon. Often these terms are used without any explanation on the assumption that they are so well known that no explanation is needed. At other times, however, it's very difficult to know what is being said without being a member of the drug culture.

One of the questions that invariably pops up whenever anyone talks about the language of marihuana is where terms like marihuana, pot, and grass came from or when they first began to be used. Unfortunately, the etymology of many of these words is lost. However, whenever possible, I have tried to provide the earliest citations for the terms that appear in this dictionary so that at least the history is documented. Many of the terms that refer to marihuana or marihuana usage also are recognized as having evolved from narcotics slang. However, only when the term clearly referred to marihuana was the entry included.

To make this dictionary more thorough, I also have included terms referring to hemp that were once well known but are now obsolete. Most of these terms refer to the use of the marihuana plant as an important source of fiber—especially in ropes used to execute people. I also have included information concerning some of the better-known people who have contributed in one way or another to the history of marihuana and concerning important events associated with the drug. Some basic information about marihuana as a plant and drug, along with some basic terms about drugs in general, also is included. Finally, an appendix is included that lists various terms for marihuana in foreign languages, along with the names and ingredients of various candies and beverages made with marihuana throughout the world.

A detailed index is provided at the end of the text that lists the dictionary entries. In addition, there are cross-references to synonyms in the text to facilitate explanation of terms. These synonyms, which are defined separately, are indicated by the symbol (*).

If readers are familiar with earlier citations of terms, if they know of other derivations for cited terms, or if they know of additional terms, they are invited to submit this information to me for possible inclusion in future editions of this book.

A
MARIHUANA
DICTIONARY

THE DICTIONARY

A

A(tom) Bomb. Cigarette made of a combination of drugs, for example, marihuana and heroin. *See also* Candy a J.
1962: "My name is Emp and I pay thirty for atom bombs." (Pritchie, *Savage Kick*, p. 24).
1965: "Sometimes marihuana cigarettes are dipped in heroin ('A-bomb') by the smoker, as one way of getting more of a 'charge' from it." (Winick, "Marihuana," p. 236).

Abuse. 1. Use of a drug for nonmedical purposes. 2. Drug usage in excess of approved medical or social practice, usually resulting in emotional or physical damage and/or antisocial behavior.

Acapulco Gold. Potent form of marihuana originating near the tropical resort town in Mexico; golden brown in color. Formerly known as Gold Leaf.*
1965: "This is a special grade of pot growing only in the vicinity of Acapulco. The color is either brownish gold or a mixture of gold and green. This grade has a potency surpassed by few of the

green varieties and usually comes at slightly higher prices or in short weight." (*Marijuana Newsletter*, January, no. 11).

1966: *Acapulco Gold.* Title of a song recorded by Rainy Daze.

1967: "The all-time supersmoke is the top cut of Mexico's vintage grass called Acapulco Gold." (*Newsweek*, July 24, p. 48).

1967: " 'Very good stuff,' he said, 'comparable to Acapulco Gold.' " (Simmons, *Marihuana*, p. 34).

1968: "Because of this 'Acapulco Gold' and 'Panama Red' have become very popular." (Bloomquist, *Marihuana*, p. 190).

1969: "Acapulco Gold . . . supposedly the all-time supersmoke of the many different varieties of marihuana tobacco." (Geller and Boas, *Drug Beat*, p. xv).

1974: *Acapulco Gold.* Title of book written by Edwin Corley.

1979: "They want to be able to drop heavy names like Acapulco Gold." (Goldman, *Grass Roots*, p. 36).

Acapulco Gold Papers. Cigarette papers made from marihuana fiber.

1974: "Their Acapulco Gold papers much improved." (*High Times*, vol. 1, no. 1, p. 5).

Acapulco Red. Like Acapulco Gold* except the color is reddish brown.

Ace. Marihuana cigarette (1930s-1940s). Term evolved by analogy with the playing card, which is the "highest" in the deck.

1938: "An ace is a single stick and sells for fifteen cents." (Berger, *New Yorker*, March 12, p. 43).

1944: "I smoke an ace and it makes me high." (Marcovitz and Myers, "Marihuana Addict," p. 384).

Action. Any activity; a "happening"; the purchase or sale of drugs. *See* Bag Action, Box Action, Grass Action, Lid Action, Pound Action, Tin Action.

Acute. Of short duration, in contrast to chronic.*

Addict. "Any individual who habitually uses any narcotic drug so as to endanger the public morals, health, safety, or welfare, or who is so far addicted to the use of narcotic drugs as to have lost the power of self-control with reference to his addiction." (*Comprehensive Drug Abuse Prevention and Control Act* of 1970). Inappropriately applied to marihuana users. *See also* Addiction.

1931: "Approximately one out of every four persons arrested in this city is addicted to mariahuana." (Fossier, "Marihuana," p. 249).

1931: "Addicts are commonly termed 'muggle heads.' " (Stanley, "Marihuana," p. 255).

1938: "The hard-working father of a family of eight was injured to the extent of a fractured skull by a marihuana addict." (Cooper, *Here's to Crime*, p. 336).

1938: "Over two hundred children under fourteen are believed to be addicted to the marihuana habit." (Walton, *Marihuana*, p. 29).

1948: "The marihuana addicts are prone to awake afterwards with a feeling of ravenous hunger." (Wolff, "Marihuana," p. 14).

1951: "We saw them serve drinks after hours and cater to fairies of all shades, female white thrill chasers, and Negro reefer addicts." (Lait and Mortimer, *Washington Confidential*, p. 71).

Addiction. A condition resulting from repeated drug use, consisting of an overpowering urge to keep using it and to get it by any means. Tendency is to increase the dosage. The condition involves both tolerance* and withdrawal symptoms following abstinence. The condition does not apply to marihuana, although marihuana users were often labeled as addicts by antimarihuana crusaders. *See also* Addict.

1952: "In the rituals of reefer addiction . . ." (Oursler and Smith, *Hooked*, p. 36).

Afghani. Hashish from Afghanistan; hash oil.*

1976: "There seem to be many different types of hash oils being marketed today . . . Afghani. . . ." (*High Times*, July, p. 16).

African Black. Potent form of hashish from Africa; blackish in color.

Airplane. *See* Jefferson Airplane.

Alcott, Louisa May (1832-1888). American novelist. Author of popular *Little Women* (1868). First (1869) American writer to use hashish as a plot device. In her short story *Perilous Play*, Alcott describes some of the effects of hashish for nineteenth-century Americans:

> "A heavenly dreaminess comes over one, in which they move as if on air. Everything is calm and lovely to them: no pain, no care, no fear of anything, and while it lasts one feels like an angel half asleep."
>
> "But if one takes too much, how then?"
>
> "Hum! Well, that's not so pleasant, unless one likes phantoms, frenzies, and a touch of nightmare, which seems to last a thousand years."

Alice B. Toklas Brownies; Hash Brownies. Cookies baked with marihuana or hashish. From Alice B. Toklas, female companion and cook for expatriate author Gertrude Stein, during the 1920s and 1930s in Paris, who used hashish in fudge recipe (*Alice B. Toklas Cookbook*, 1929).

Recipe inspired movie, *I Love You, Alice B. Toklas*, about effects of brownies baked with marihuana.

1969: "I was warned to be careful if I mixed pot in food—Alice B. Toklas brownies or 'apple turn-on.'" (*Time*, September 26, p. 73).

1976: "If grass is smoked or baked in the oven (Alice B. Toklas Brownies)...." (*High Times*, May, p. 13).

All right on the hemp. An expression current before the American Civil War meaning "to be held accountable." Equivalent to modern expression, "put your money where your mouth is." During the pre-Civil War era, it literally meant that you were willing to hang someone as proof of your conviction that you were right and he was wrong. Hanging ropes at that time were made of hemp—the fiber of the marihuana plant—hence the expression. *See* Hemp.

1857: "In the northern districts, the piece of hemp was the more customary mark of those who were ready to use the halter in proof of the soundness of their views. 'Neither give nor take quarter,' and 'all right on the hemp' were their two pass words." (Gladstone, *Englishman in Kansas*, pp. 255-56).

Amok, Amuck. Uncontrollable behavior, generally involving violence. "To run amok" means to run about in a frenzy, attacking everyone encountered. Phrase originated in Malaya and was associated with marihuana usage.

1893-1894: "The Inspector-General of Police in the Central Provinces states that 'running amok' is always the result of excessive indulgence in hemp drugs; but under cross-examination he says: 'I have never had experience of such a case. I only state what I have heard.'" (*India Hemp Drugs Commission Report*, pp. 258-59).

1936: "In Malay, where it is eaten as hashish, the murderous frenzy in which the native dashes with a weapon into a crowd screaming: 'Amok! Amok!' (Kill! Kill!) is due to the drug, according to some travelers. Our common expression 'to run amuck' is derived from this source." (Wolf, *Popular Science Monthly*, p. 119).

Amorphia. California-based lobbying group for legalization of marihuana. Founded in 1969 by Dr. Michael Aldrich, the membership primarily was made up of marihuana users. The group succeeded in placing a referendum to legalize marihuana on the California ballot in 1972 (not passed). The group disappeared after 1974.

Amotivational Syndrome. Term coined to describe a loss of interest in conventional goals as a result of chronic marihuana use. *See also* Canabinomania.

1969: "Scientists are now trying to assess what some call the 'amotivational syndrome.' " (*Newsweek*, April 21, p. 110).
1969: "The regular use of marihuana may be followed by an 'amotivational syndrome.' " (*Time*, July 25, p. 65).

Angola Black. Potent marihuana from Angola; dark in color.

Ann Arbor Ordinance. First (1971) local law in the United States decriminalizing marihuana use from a felony* offense to a misdemeanor*
with a maximum sentence of ninety days in jail and/or a $100 fine.

Anslinger, Harry Jacob (1892-1975). Commissioner of the Federal
Bureau of Narcotics* (1930-1962). Anslinger is the law enforcement
official most closely linked with antimarihuana laws in America. He
was the driving force behind the enactment of the Marihuana Tax Act
of 1937* and an advocate of strong antidrug laws and stiff penalties
for violation. Prone to exaggeration, hyperbole, and distortions when
discussing marihuana, and calling it "as dangerous as a coiled rattle-
snake and twice as deadly," he said, "If the hideous monster Franken-
stein came face to face with the monster marihuana he would drop
dead of fright." Anslinger retired as bureau chief in 1962 but served
as U.S. representative on the United Nations International Narcotics
Control Board until 1970.

Antiparaphernalia Law. Law banning the sale of paraphernalia associated with drug taking, including marihuana, for example, marihuana cigarette papers. The first (1977) statewide law was passed in
Indiana. *See* Head Shop.

Anywhere. Possessing or smoking marihuana.
1953: "Are you anywhere?" (Burroughs, *Junkie*, p. 14).

Aphrodisiac. Substance that increases libido. It does so by reducing
inhibitions or increasing local genital irritation. Marihuana is often
regarded as such.
1939: ". . . reefers, i.e., the aphrodisiac made from the crushed leaves
and seeds of the marihuana plant." (*Fortune*, July, p. 60).
1949: "Marihuana can be a strong aphrodisiac and for its users there
is usually no such thing as normal sex relations." (Wilson,
Collier's, June 4, p. 53).

Arabian Nights (also known as Thousand and One Nights). Collection
of stories from Arab-speaking countries, some of which are more than
a thousand years old. These stories tell of daily life in Arab countries,
and some refer to hashish and its effects, especially on sexuality. The

stories were the first introduction to hashish and its effects for most
Europeans.

> "Know that the most delicious thing that my ear has ever heard, O my young
> lord, is this story that came to me of a hashish eater among hashish eaters."
> (from *Tale of the Hashish Eater*).

> "There was once, my lord, crown of my head, a man in a certain city who
> was a fisherman by trade and a hashish eater by occupation." (from *Tale of
> the Two Hashish Eaters*).

Ashes. Marihuana.

Assassins. Name given to a terrorist group operating during the eleventh
through thirteenth centuries in the Middle East. The group was founded
around A.D. 1050 by Hasan-ibn Sabah, known to the Crusaders as the
"Old Man of the Mountain." Their base of operations was initially
Persia, but their influence spread as far as Syria. The group allegedly
used hashish. By association, hashish became identified with violence
and murder by Westerners.

1936: "(The word) 'assassin' has two explanations, but either demon-
strates the menace of Indian hemp. According to one version,
members of a band of Persian terrorists committed their worst
atrocities while under the influence of hashish. In the other version, Saracens who opposed the Crusaders were said to employ
the services of hashish addicts to secure secret murders of the
leaders of the Crusades. In both versions, the murderers were
known as 'haschischin.' " (Wolf, *Popular Science Magazine*,
p. 14).

1937: "The members were confirmed users of hashish, or marihuana,
and it is from the Arab 'hashashin' that we have the English
word 'assassin.' " (Anslinger, *American Magazine*, p. 9).

At. Where something is taking place. "Where's it at? Where's the pot
party?"

Atharva Veda. Religious text from India dating back to 2,000-1,400 B.C.
containing earliest written reference to marihuana (as "bhanga").

Aubert-Roche, Louis (1808-1878). French physician. Aubert-Roche
practiced medicine in Egypt between 1834-1838. He wrote "The Use
of Hashish in the Treatment of the Plague" (1840), which dealt with
beneficial effects of hashish in the treatment of typhus.

Aunt Mary. Marihuana.

Ayurvedic. Traditional medical system of India that uses marihuana to treat various problems such as diarrhea, cholera, tetanus, insomnia, loss of appetite, and malaria.

B

B(ee), Bag. 1. Drug container. *See* Baggie, Dime Bag, Nickel Bag.
2. Quantity of marihuana that could fit into a penny matchbox.
3. Activity, personal interests, obsessions.
1967: "An ounce of marihuana has around five B's to it." (Rosevear, *Pot*, p. 28).

Baby. Marihuana.
1960: "He call it 'baby.' " (Southern, "Red Dirt Marihuana," p. 219).

Bad. 1. Unpleasant, painful. *See* Bad Head, Bad Scene, Bad Trip.
2. Used as an understatement or reversal of real intent, meaning good, excellent.

Bad Head. Mentally confused as a result of using marihuana or other drugs.

Bad Scene. Unpleasant situation.

Bad Trip. Unpleasant drug reaction, for example, panic and anxiety. Generally associated with LSD, but also with other drugs, such as marihuana.

Bag Action. Purchase of a bag of marihuana. *See* Baggie.
1967: "Buying a small container might be called 'bag action.' " (Rosevear, *Pot*, p. 28).

Baggie. Plastic sandwich bag containing about an ounce of marihuana.
1967: ". . . packaged the ounces in baggies." (Ric, *Esquire*, p. 28).

Bale of Hay. Unspecified quantity of marihuana.
1969: "Bale of Hay . . . a bulky amount of marihuana, so-called be-
        cause it is difficult to flush down the toilet—the usual way to
get rid of it in case of emergency." (Geller and Boas, *Drug Beat*, p. xv)

Balloon Room. Place where marihuana is smoked.
1960: "Balloon room." (Wentworth and Flexner, *Dictionary*, p. 17).

Balloon room without a parachute. A marihuana pad* where all the marihuana is gone.

Bambalacha. Marihuana, hashish.
1943: "Marihuana may be called . . . bambalacha." (*Time*, July 19, p. 54).
1951: "Bambalacha." (Bouquet, *Bulletin on Narcotics*, p. 32).
1974: "Bambalacha encourages spontaneity." (Isyurhash and Rusoff, *Gourmet*, p. 11).

Bambalacha Rambler. Marihuana smoker.
1959: "Bambalacha rambler." (Schmidt, *Narcotics*, p. 9).

Bambu. Brand of cigarette paper for smoking marihuana. Most popular brand among the beatniks of the 1950s.

Bambu Case. Metal container for marihuana cigarette paper.

Bammies, Bams. Low-potency marihuana cigarettes.
1956: "Cheap bammies you can pick up at about three for a quarter." (Hunter, *Second Ending*, p. 221).
1959: "Bams." (Murtagh and Harris, *Who Live in Shadows*, p. 199).

Banana Smoking. *See* Mellow Yellow.

Bang. 1. Morphine injection. 2. Smoke marihuana. 3. Marihuana, from the Indian term, bhang; *see* appendix.
1935: "Bang: Marihuana." (Pollock, *Underworld Speaks*, p. 5).
1950: "Bang: To smoke a cigarette of marihuana." (Goldin, *Dictionary*, p. 22).

Bar. Compressed block of marihuana stuck together with sugar, honey, or Coca-Cola. *See also* Sugared.
1967: "Bar. . . . An imported quantity of marihuana pressed into a block." (Rosevear, *Pot*, p. 155).

Bash. Good time; a party; a spree.

Baudelaire, Charles (1821-1861). French poet and writer. Baudelaire was a member of the Hashish Club (Club des Haschischins). Although he rarely used hashish himself, his *Artificial Paradises (Les Paradis Artificiels)*, published in 1858, contains often-quoted and lyric descriptions of the hashish experience. Although he died of syphilis, his death was attributed to overindulgence in hashish.

> "It is right, then, that sophisticated persons, and also ignorant persons who are eager to make acquaintance with unusual delights, should be clearly

told that they will find in hashish nothing miraculous, absolutely nothing but an exaggeration of the natural. The brain and organism on which hashish operates will produce only the normal phenomena peculiar to the individual—increased admittedly, in number and force, but always faithful to their origin. A man will never escape from his destined physical and moral temperament: hashish will be a mirror of his impression and private thoughts—a magnifying mirror, it is true, but only a mirror."

Be in tweeds. Smoke marihuana.

Be sent. Satisfied and in a stupor from smoking marihuana.

Beam Test. Forensic test for detecting presence of marihuana in unknown material. The test material is mixed with alcohol and potassium hydroxide. If marihuana is present, the mixture turns purple. This test is no longer used due to lack of its specificity.

Beaming. Intoxicated; high.

Beat Pad. Place where low-potency marihuana is sold (1930s-1940s).
1938: "Tea pads where inferior cigarettes are sold are beat pads."
        (Berger, *New Yorker*, March 12, p. 47).

Beat the weeds. Smoke marihuana.
1970: "Beat the weeds." (*Current Slang*, vol. 4, no. 2, p. 4).

Beaten. Unable to function as a result of chronic, excessive marihuana use. *See also* Brain burned, Wasted.

Bee. *See* B(ee), Bag.

Belted. Intoxicated; high.

Bending the head. Smoking marihuana.

Bent. Under the influence of marihuana; high.
Bent out of shape. 1. Angry; disgruntled. 2. Intoxicated; high.

Bethesda Gold. Marihuana, not very potent.
1969: ". . . despite the magnitude of 'Tennessee blue' and 'Bethesda gold,'. . . ." (*Time*, September 26, p. 69).

Bhang. Marihuana; *see* appendix.

Big John. Police officer.

Bim. Police officer.

Birdwood. Marihuana (1940s).

Bit. Personal interests; activity.

Bite one's lips. Smoke marihuana.
1959: "Bite one's lips." (Schmidt, *Narcotics*, p. 17).

Black. Potent hashish. Usually not sold for profit but instead used by dealers* for their own pleasure.
1975: "The Congo has turned in a credible harvest of potent black."
      (*High Times*, October, p. 44).
1976: "We rolled up a joint of black and sat him on his ass." (Sorfleet,
      "Dealing," p. 146).

Black Columbus. Marihuana.

Black Gold. Potent marihuana.
1946: ". . . black gold . . . an expensive hemp of great strength be-
      lieved to be imported from Mexico or India." (Charen and
      Perelman, "Marihuana Addicts," p. 678).

Black Gungeon, Gunion. Potent marihuana, viscous and black colored.
Derived from the Jamaican term *ganja*, which in turn originates from
Indian term *ganja; see* appendix.
1969: "I got 'black gunion,' baby." (Iceberg Slim, *Pimp*, p. 181).
1972: "Black Gungeon." (Folb, *Black Argot*, p. 89).

Black Hash. Hashish; black in color. *See* Black.

Black Mo, Moat, Mold, Mole, Monte, Mota. 1. Potent marihuana.
2. Marihuana mixed with sugar or honey. Popular in the 1940s as
muta, * which is a Mexican term for marihuana; *see* appendix.
1972: "Black Mo." (Folb, *Black Argot*, p. 90).

Black Oil. Hash oil.*
1977: ". . . the commercial mass-produced, black oil from Nepal,
      Lebanon and Morocco . . ." (*High Times*, February, p. 68).

Black Russian. Hashish from Russia; black in color.

Black and White. Police car.

Blanco y Negro. Brand of marihuana cigarette papers, literally "black
and white." *See also* Salt and Pepper.

Blank. Low-potency marihuana.

Blanket. Papers for making marihuana cigarettes.
1935: "Blanket: Cigarette paper." (Pollock, *Underworld Speaks*, p. 5).

Blast. 1. Rapid, strong effect from smoking marihuana. Originally from
narcotics slang (1930s). 2. To smoke marihuana.

1943: "The viper may then quietly blast the weed." (*Time*, July 19, p. 54).

1944: "I straightened up and blasted another one." (Marcovitz and Myers, "Marihuana Addict," p. 384).

1955: "It was the strangeness of Americans and Mexicans blasting together in the desert." (Kerouac, *Road*, p. 283).

1957: "Georgette blasted with a vengeance." (Selby, *Last Exit*, p. 38).

1962: "Howie and I blasted two joints." (Pritchie, *Savage Kick*, p. 14).

Blast a joint, reefers, stick, weed. Smoke marihuana. *See* Blast.

1971: "Vic and I were blasting this joint." (Jones and Chilton, *Louis*, p. 113).

Blast Mary Jane to Kingdom Come. To smoke marihuana cigarettes one after another.

1959: "Blast . . . come." (Schmidt, *Narcotics*, p. 17).

Blast party. Party where marihuana is smoked. *See also* Pot Party.

1970: "Blast party." (Cromwell, *Slang*, p. 77).

Blasted. Under the influence of marihuana; intoxicated; high.*

Blind. Very high.* *See* Wasted, Wrecked.

Blind Munchies. Overwhelming craving for any kind of food after smoking marihuana.

Blitzed. Under the influence of marihuana; very high.*

Block. A kilogram (2.2 pounds) of marihuana.

1966: "The connection brings out the grass tightly pressed into one pound blocks." (*Village Voice*, December 1, p. 20).

Blocked. Under the influence of marihuana; high.*

1968: "Blocked." (Dawtry, *Drug Abuse*, p. 87).

Blond. Hashish from Lebanon or Morocco. Not as potent as Black.*

Blow. 1. To smoke marihuana. 2. To snort heroin or cocaine.

1944: "I want to rush in a subway train again and visit a pad and blow some hemp once more." (Marcovitz and Myers, "Marihuana Addict," p. 391).

1953: "We're all out of charge so I'll dash in and get some and we'll blow one more." (Wallop, *Night Light*, p. 136).

1960: "Sniffing and popping replaced blowing and lighting up or turning on, though the latter two might be used interchangeably." (De Mexico, *Marijuana Girl*, p. 118).

1968: "I blew some pot in the shit house." (Thomas, *Mean Streets*, p. 221).

1969: "Blow a stick." (Williams, *Narcotics*, p. 109).

1969: "Many adults who 'blow' pot are overeager to stay young." (*Time*, September 26, p. 69).

1971: "We'd get up in the morning . . . and blow a couple of joints each." (Hall, *Heads*, p. 38).

Blow Gage, Grass, Hay, Hemp, a Joint, a Reefer, a Stick, Tea. To smoke marihuana.

Blow One's Cool. To lose self-control; become angry.

Blow One's Mind. 1. To become high* on marihuana. 2. To alter consciousness. 3. To lose sanity.

Blow One's Top. 1. To become high* on marihuana. 2. To become angry.

1953: "The weed available in the U.S. is evidently not strong enough to blow your top." (Burroughs, *Junkie*, p. 38).

Blowtop. Marihuana user.

1948: "Some blowtop pulled this, all right." (Schwartz, *Blowtop*, p. 57).

Blue Cheese. Hashish.

Blue de Hue. Marihuana. Term used by American soldiers in Vietnam.

Blue Fascist. Police officer.

Blue Sage. Marihuana (1930s-1940s).

1943: "Marihuana may be called . . . blue sage." (*Time*, July 19, p. 54).

Blue Sky Blond. Potent marihuana from Colombia.

BNDD. Bureau of Narcotics and Dangerous Drugs.

Bo Bo. Marihuana.

Bo Bo Bush. Marihuana.

1936: "Bo bo bush." (Maurer, "Argot of Underworld," p. 119).

1942: "Bo bo bush." (Berrey and Bark, *Thesaurus*, p. 474).

1966: "Bo bo bush." (Siragusa, *Trail of the Poppy*, p. 224).

1969: "Bo bo bush." (Geller and Boas, *Drug Beat*, p. xviii).

Bo Bo Jockey. Marihuana user.

1959: "Bo bo jockey." (Schmidt, *Narcotics*, p. 19).

Bogart a joint. To salivate on or not pass a marihuana cigarette to another smoker quickly enough. Derived from dangling cigarette associated with actor Humphrey Bogart.

1971: "One of the girls bogarts the joint." (Coyote Man, *Buzz*, p. 86).
1978: "If you bogart a joint, you probably deserve to die." (*Playboy*, September, p. 164).

Boggs, H. Congressman and chairman of Ways and Means Subcommittee on Narcotics. Proponent of stiff penalties for violation of drug laws to eliminate drug traffic including marihuana. *See* Boggs Act.

Boggs Act. 1951 law increasing severity of penalties for violation of drug laws. First-time penalties for violation of marihuana laws were made the same as those for violation of narcotics laws. This act introduced minimum mandatory jail sentences for first offenses. It led to the passage of "Little Boggs Acts"—state laws mandating harsh penalties for violation of drug laws including lengthy minimum sentences for first offenses and maximum sentences and sometimes death penalty for subsequent convictions.

Bomb, Bomber. Thick marihuana cigarette.
1952: "Bomber: giant size marihuana cigarette." (Lannoy and Masterson, "Hophead Jargon," p. 24).
1955: "Victor proceeded to roll the biggest bomber anyone had ever seen." (Kerouac, *Road*, p. 283).
1956: "You can get the better muggles, the bombers, for about a dollar each." (Hunter, *Second Ending*, p. 221).
1959: "They were in great big bombers, man, like king size." (Lipton, *Holy Barbarians*, p. 187).
1968: "It was a king sized bomber." (Thomas, *Mean Streets*, p. 65).
1969: "The bomber in her hand was now a roach." (Iceberg Slim, *Pimp*, p. 182).
1971: "One cat pulled out a big 'bomber.' " (Jones and Chilton, *Louis*, p. 116).
1974: "Bombers can be as large as two feet." (Isyurhash and Rusoff, *Gourmet*, p. 53).
1979: "He passes me a fuming bomber." (Goldman, *Grass Roots*, p. 23).

Bombed. Under the influence of marihuana; very high.*
1968: "They'd be out fighting at night and during the day they'd get bombed on grass." (Gross, *Flower People*, p. 11).

Bong. Pipe in which smoker draws from stem attached to upper part of bowl. The bowl fills with smoke and provides a sustained, concentrated flow of smoke allowing smoker to inhale large amounts of smoke and thereby produce a more intense effect. Popular device in

Asia. Introduced to America by GIs returning from Vietnam circa
1970.

1971: "Originally from Thailand, the Bong has now come to America."
(*Marihuana Review*, vol. 1, no. 6, p. 18).

1975: "I want to enjoy the true Bong Experience." (*High Times*,
August, p. 11).

Boo, Bu. Marihuana.

1967: "Boo." (Polsky, *Hustlers*, p. 165).

1967: "He's got to call it 'weed' and 'boo.' " (Ric, *Esquire*, September, p. 190).

1968: "Boo." (Gross, *Flower People*, p. 171).

1979: "They called it 'tea,' 'boo,' 'grass,' and 'pot.' " (Goldman, *Grass
Roots*, p. 113).

Boo Hoo. Priest in Neo-American Church who uses marihuana and
other drugs as a religious sacrament.

1976: "Art Kleps, Chief Boo Hoo, Neo-American Church." (*High
Times*, March, p. 21).

Boo Reefer. Marihuana cigarette.

1972: Boo reefer: marihuana cigarette. (Claerbaut, *Black Jargon*, p. 58).

Boon. Wooden part of the stalk of the marihuana plant.

Booster stick. Tobacco cigarette to which marihuana extract has been
added.

1973: Booster stick: "An ordinary cigarette, the tip of which is dipped
in a concentrated essence of marihuana preserved in alcohol."
(Maurer, *Narcotics*, p. 391).

Boot. Kicks; thrills; excitement.

1956: "What happens when you no longer get a boot from it?"
(Hunter, *Second Ending*, p. 251.)

Bopper. Adolescent. *See* Teeny-bopper.

Boreroom Beater. Marihuana smoker.

1955: "Boreroom beater." (Braddy, "Narcotic Argot," p. 86).

Bounce the goof balls. To smoke marihuana cigarettes.

1959: Bounce the goof balls: "To smoke marihuana." (Schmidt, *Narcotics*, p. 19).

Box. *See* B(ee), Bag.

Boxed. High*; stoned.*

1967: "Boxed." (Rosevear, *Pot*, p. 156).

Boy. 1. Heroin. 2. Marihuana.
1955: "Boy." (Braddy, "Narcotic Argot," p. 86).

Bract. Greenish sheath covering marihuana seeds.

Brain burned. Very intoxicated from smoking marihuana. No longer able to function as a result of chronic marihuana or other drug use.

Bread. Money.

Break. To separate marihuana fibers from the stalk. Also, the machine that did the separation.

Break a stick. To smoke marihuana.
1959: Break a stick: To smoke a marihuana cigarette. (Schmidt, *Narcotics*, p. 20).

Breckenridge Green. Low-potency marihuana from Kentucky.

Brick. Kilogram of marihuana compressed into the shape of a brick.
1967: "When I came back, I started to hustle pot. Light stuff, here and there a few bricks." (Thomas, *Mean Streets*, p. 57).
1967: ". . . packs the trunk of his new car with kilo bricks." (*Look*, August 18, p. 12).

Bridge. A device to hold a burning marihuana cigarette butt. *See* Roach Clip, Jefferson Airplane.
1955: "Bridge: A holder for marihuana cigarettes." (Braddy, "Narcotic Argot," p. 86).

Brifo. Marihuana. Variation of grifo. *See* Greefa.
1937: "A number of other names are also used such as . . . 'brifo.' " (Weber, "Mary Warner," p. 77).

Bring down. To calm someone who has become agitated from smoking marihuana; to return someone to an unintoxicated state.
1938: "When a customer gets ready to 'cut out' [leave] Chippy 'brings him down' with milk." (Berger, *New Yorker*, March 12, p. 47).
1962: "They were both too high for a hot afternoon like this one and stopped off for lunch to bring themselves down." (Pritchie, *Savage Kick*, p. 68).

Broccoli. Marihuana.
1969: "Marihuana (. . . 'broccoli' . . .) is their favorite preparation." (*Time*, September 26, p. 68).

Broom Rape *(Orobanche ramosa).* Only parasite to which the marihuana plant is vulnerable.

Bu. *See* Boo.

Budda, Buddha Sticks. Marihuana. *See* Thai Sticks.

Bugged. 1. Bothered; pestered; harassed. 2. Initiated into the use of marihuana.

Bull. Police officer.

Bull Horror. Paranoia* concerning arrest. Individual thinks everyone is a police officer and is disturbed by the slightest sound.
1939: "Bull horrors." (De Leeuw, *Flower*, p. 229).

Bull Jive. Marihuana adulterated with oregano, catnip, or other impotent material.

Bum Rap. Arrested or convicted when innocent.

Bum Trip. Unpleasant experience from smoking marihuana, for example, anxiety, panic, paranoia.*
Bummer. Any unpleasant experience; a sense of depression or paranoia* resulting from drug use. *See* Bum Trip.

Bunk. Low-potency marihuana.

Burn an Indian. 1. To smoke marihuana. 2. Become addicted to marihuana.
1959: "Burn an Indian." (Schmidt, *Narcotics*, p. 22).

Burn Artist. Dishonest drug seller.
1978: "No burn artist would wrap a package like this." (*High Times*, July, p. 79).

Burn the Hay. Smoke marihuana.

Burned. 1. Cheated by buying a phony drug, adulterated marihuana, or by not receiving the drug for payment. 2. Recognized; undercover officer's identity exposed.
1961: "She started burning us on a few details." (Hughes, *Fantastic Lodge*, p. 138).
1966: ". . . to avoid the danger of being robbed or 'burned.' " (*Village Voice*, December 1, p. 20).
1971: "They have been getting burned on a lot of stuff." (Hall, *Heads*, p. 40).
1971: "Did you ever get burned on bad reefer?" (Woodley, *Dealer*, p. 124).

Burned Out. 1. Unable to function; deteriorated physically and mentally from marihuana or other drug use; unaware of surroundings; inability to concentrate from prolonged, heavy use of marihuana. 2. Given up using marihuana.

Burnies. 1. Marihuana cigarettes. 2. Partially smoked marihuana cigarettes.
1949: "Burnie." (Monteleone, *Criminal Slang*, p. 39).
1952: "Burnie." (Lannoy and Masterson, "Hophead Jargon," p. 24).

Bush. Marihuana. *See also* Bo Bo Bush.
1965: "Marijuana—which besides pot, also goes under the names of Mary jane, grass, weed, hay, bush, tea, hemp, stuff, and it among others. . . ." (*New York Post*, December 3, p. 45).
1968: "Where can I buy some bush?" (U. California, *Folklore*, p. 416).
1972: "What is commonly referred to as marijuana (often called 'grass', 'pot', 'weed(s)', 'bush', 'tea', 'reefer', 'boo', 'Mary Jane' or the more general 'dope' or 'shit'). . . ." (*Le Dain Commission*, p. 11).
1974: ". . . attempting to bring nine-and-a-half tons of Jamaican bush up the small west Florida waterway. . . ." (*High Times*, vol. 1, no. 1, p. 15).

Bush Tea. Tea made with marihuana.

Bushwacker. Marihuana smoker.
1959: "Bushwacker." (Schmidt, *Narcotics*, p. 22).

Bust. 1. Smoke marihuana. 2. Arrest; *see* Busted.
1956: "You can bust a joint right on the street." (Hunter, *Second Ending*, p. 94).

Busted. Arrested.
1938: " 'Bust' is Harlem for a raid." (Berger, *New Yorker*, March 12, p. 48).
1952: "They busted Magoo." (Mandell, *Flee the Angry Strangers*, p. 224).
1955: "The next day I got busted/As I walked out of the door." (Braddy, "Anonymous Verses," p. 131).
1956: "You got busted you say." (Duke, *Sideman*, p. 274).
1959: "Only a cat is 'busted'; a square is arrested." (Lipton, *Holy Barbarians*, p. 315).

Buster. Federal narcotics officer.

Butter Flower. Marihuana.

Buy. Purchase marihuana.

Buzz. 1. Early sensations as the effects of marihuana begin to be felt.
2. Mild, euphoric feeling from smoking marihuana. 3. Intoxicated.
4. To buy marihuana. *See also* Rolling Buzz.
1952: "Buzz." (Lannoy and Masterson, "Hophead Jargon," p. 24).
1955: "I smoked some more and got a buzz." (Braddy, "Anonymous
        Verses," p. 130).
1960: *Where the buzz is*
        There the fuzz is
        Coming through the door."
        (Trocchi, *Cain's Book*, p. 108).
1962: "He had a slight buzz himself from the three roaches he had
        smoked." (Pritchie, *Savage Kick*, p. 13).
1967: ". . . a three or four hour buzz referred to in the vernacular as
        being stoned." (Brown, *Hippies*, p. 182).

C

Cache. Hidden supply of marihuana or other drugs. *See also* Stache.
1976: ". . . a really elegant way to keep your cache intact." (*High
        Times*, March, p. 90).
1980: "Once I found a VC cache which contained some marijuana."
        (Novak, *High Culture*, p. 170).

Cam (Cambodian) Red. Reddish-brown marihuana from Cambodia;
very potent.
1968: "GIs can score packets of American filter tips loaded with Cam-
        bodian Red." (*Marihuana Review*, vol. 1, no. 1, p. 4).

Cambodian Trip Weed. Potent marihuana from Cambodia; black in
color. *See* Trip.

Can. One or two ounces of marihuana in a can. Term originated from
Prince Albert tobacco cans in which marihuana was commonly sold in
the 1930s and 1940s.
1967: ". . . five 'cans' (he wouldn't call it ounces)." (Ric, *Esquire*, Sep-
        tember, p. 190).
1969: "I want a sixteenth of 'girl' and a can of reefer." (Iceberg Slim,
        Pimp, p. 133).

Can Action. Buying or selling a can of marihuana.
1968: "Can action." (Rosevear, *Pot*, p. 28).

Can you do me some good? Can you sell me marihuana or other drugs? 1955: "Can you do me some good?" (Braddy, "Narcotic Argot," p. 86).

Canabinomania. Loss of interest in everyday activities resulting from the use of marihuana. *See also* Amotivational Syndrome.
1933: "After the chronic use of marihuana 'Canabinomania' develops in which many persons, especially psychopathic, leads to a loss of mental activity, accompanied by general dullness and indolence, like that of chronic alcoholics or opium eaters." (Hayes and Bowery, "Marihuana," p. 1089-90).

Canadian Black. Black-colored marihuana from Canada.

Cancelled Stick. 1. Tobacco cigarette emptied of its tobacco and replaced with marihuana. 2. Low-potency marihuana.
1969: "Cancelled stick." (Geller and Boas, *Drug Beat*, p. xvi).

Candy. 1. Hashish. 2. Cocaine. 3. Gum opium.
1939: "Candy: Hashish." (Housley, *Dictionary*, p. 11).

Candy a J. To add another potent drug, for example, heroin, to a marihuana cigarette. *See* A(tom) Bomb.

Candy Jag. Craving for sweets after smoking marihuana. *See* Munchies.

Cannabicae. Botanical family to which cannabis is assigned.

Cannabinoids. Characteristic group of chemicals present in cannabis. As of 1980, sixty-one cannabinoids had been identified in marihuana. Among the most frequently mentioned are:

Delta-9-tetrahydrocannabinol	THC
Delta-8-tetrahydrocannabinol	THC
Cannabinolic acid	CBNA
Cannabinol	CBN
Cannabidiolic	CBDA
Cannabidiol	CBD
Cannabigerolic acid	CBGA
Cannabigerol	CBG
Cannabichromenic acid	CBCA
Cannabichromene	CBC
Cannabigerolic acid monomethylether	CBGM
Cannabigerol monomethylether	CBGM
Cannabicyclol	CBL
Cannabidivarin	CBV
Cannabidilic acid monomethylether	CBDAM
Cannabidivarinic acid	CBVA

Cannabis. Herb from which marihuana, hashish, and the like are obtained. Cannabis is a polytypic species of the *Cannabicae** family, which includes *Cannabis sativa,** *Cannabis indica,** and *Cannabis ruderalis.** It has been cultivated in Asia since ancient times.

Cannabis is an annual plant that grows as much as two feet a week during its peak growing period and attains heights up to eighteen feet at maturity. Seeds germinate in less than one week. Cannabis is dioecious, which means that the male and female sex organs are not found on the same plant, that is, there are distinct male and female plants. Pollination occurs by wind, since insects such as the bee are not attracted to the flowers. Male plants mature before the females and shed their pollen before they die. This shedding occurs just about the time the females come into their maturity. To prevent this pollination, male plants are pulled as soon as they can be identified. Once pollinated, resin production decreases considerably.

The resin contains the psychoactive material characteristic of cannabis. Resin is produced by structures on the leaf called trichomes.* Other parts of the resin-storing and protecting apparatus are the sessile glands* and the cysolithic hairs.* Both male and female plants produce resin. The potency of the resin is equivalent; the only difference is that the female produces more.

Cannabis is one of the oldest plants cultivated by man. Besides being used for its psychoactive effects, which derive from its principle psychoactive ingredient, delta-9-THC, the stem is the source of fiber known as hemp,* used to make rope, twine, cloth, bags, sacks, sailcloth, carpets, caulking, and many other products, and the seeds have been used as food for both men and birds. The oil within the seeds has also been used as a base for paints, varnishes, lacquers, and soap.

The psychoactive potency of marihuana depends on the concentration of delta-9-THC produced by the plant and is determined by genetic factors. Quantity of resin is also determined by climatic factors. Seeds from Afghanistan grown in the United States yield plants with the same potency THC as those grown in Afghanistan. However, the amount of THC will not be as great.

Cannabis grown for its fiber contains very little THC (less than 0.5 percent) but has a high cannabidiol (CBD) content, whereas that grown for its psychoactive effects may contain upward of 20 percent THC and very little CBD.

Cannabis indica. Marihuana plant originating in India, literally "Indian cane." *Cannabis indica* was identified in 1783 by French naturalist Lamarck,* as distinct from *Cannabis sativa** because of sativa's woodier stem, shorter height (about four feet), denser branching, and the greater strength of its psychoactive properties.

Cannabis ruderalis. Species of cannabis occurring in wild state in Central Asia. Differs from *C. indica* and *sativa* in being much smaller (one to two feet), having fewer branches, shorter leaves, and smaller seeds. It was identified as a distinct species of cannabis in 1924 by Russian botanist Janischewsky.

Cannabis sativa. Literally "cultivated cane." This botanical name was proposed in 1753 by Swedish botanist Carolus Linnaeus* in his book, *Species Plantarum*. The term was taken from an earlier text written in 1623 by botanist Berlu. The term derived from *cana* (Sanskrit) meaning "cane" or "reed," *bios* (Greek) meaning "bow," and *sativa* (Latin) meaning "cultivated."

Cannabinism. Psychosis resulting from marihuana usage.
1938: "Excessive use results in what is known as cannabinism."
     (Yawger, "Marihuana," p. 353).

Canned Goods. Any drug, including marihuana. From the selling of marihuana in Prince Albert cans. *See* Can.
1935: "Canned goods: marihuana." (Pollock, *Underworld Speaks*, p. 7).

Cap. 1. Purchase marihuana or other drugs. *See* Cop. 2. To open a drug.
1955: "I capped some more pot." (Braddy, "Anonymous Verses,"
     p. 130).

Cap Out. To become drowsy or sleepy from taking marihuana.
1972: "Cap out." (Folb, *Black Argot*, p. 8).

Carboxylation. Chemical conversion of inactive cannabinoid* acids into active substances when heated.

Carburetor. Tube with one or more holes in side. A cigarette is placed in one end and inhaled through the other with the holes on the side covered. When the tube is filled, the holes on the side are uncovered; this causes smoke to be drawn forcefully into the lungs. Same as shotgun.*
1966: "Another puff, this one not quite as long, then a series of short
     ones, carbureting the air, sucking at it noisily." (Farina, *Been
     Down So Long*, p. 34).
1976: "People are using more carburetors today, whereas seven or
     eight years ago, they didn't have carburetors." (*High Times*,
     May, p. 21).

Carrying. Possessing marihuana.

Cartucho. Package of marihuana cigarettes (Chicano), literally "cartridge."
1955: "Cartucho." (Braddy, "Narcotic Argot," p. 86).

Cat. A member of the "in-group."
1959: "Cat: The swinging, sex-free, footloose, nocturnal, uninhibited, nonconformist genus of the human race." (Lipton, *Holy Barbarians*, p. 315).

Catnip. Herb mixed with marihuana to increase its bulk so that more money can be charged. Sometimes sold as marihuana to naive buyer. *See* Burned.
1959: ". . . make a meet to sell him some 'pod' as he calls it, thinking, 'I'll catnip the jerk.' " (Burroughs, *Naked Lunch*, p. 4).

Cat-tail. Marihuana cigarette.

Charge. 1. Originally the reaction to narcotics. 2. Marihuana. 3. High*; intoxicated.
1944: "Charge is marihuana." (Burley, *Original Handbook*, p. 52).
1952: "It's only jive, but it's good charge." (Mandell, *Flee the Angry Strangers*, p. 162).
1953: "Smoke charge—okay. But once you get on that needle, man, you're gone." (Wallop, *Night Light*, p. 147).
1956: "Suppose it did take two joints after a while to bring on any sort of charge." (Hunter, *Second Ending*, p. 250).
1956: "Tell me about the night you first smoked charge." (Thorpe, *Hooked*, p. 6).
1960: "He call it charge." (Southern, "Red Dirt Marihuana," p. 61).
1960: "There's only one thing charge does for you." (De Mexico, *Marijuana Girl*, p. 46).

Cheeo. Marihuana seeds.
1971: "Cheeo." (Maurer, *Narcotics*, p. 396).

Cherry Leb. Hash oil* from Lebanon.
1976: "There seem to be many different types of hash oils being marketed today . . . cherry Leb. . . ." (*High Times*, July, p. 16).

Chiba Chiba. Potent marihuana.
1971: "Chiba-chiba." (*Marihuana Review*, vol. 1, no. 8, p. 24).
1974: "Colombian, small gold colitas buds. The original chiba-chiba." (*High Times*, vol. 1, no. 2, p. 38).

Chicago Black. Potent marihuana; black colored.

Chicago Green. Potent marihuana; green colored.

Chicharra. Mixture of marihuana and tobacco.
1970: "Chicarra." (Brennan, *Drugs*, p. 60).

Chill. To refuse to sell marihuana or any drugs to a prospective buyer.

Chillum. Cone-shaped pipe for smoking marihuana. Marihuana is packed into the top part of the cone and is covered with a cloth. The bottom of cone is held in hand and smoke is inhaled from cupped hands.

Chira. Marihuana. From *charas; see* appendix.

Chlorodyne. Stomach remedy manufactured by Squibb Co., in the late nineteenth and early twentieth century, that contained marihuana.

Chocolate. Hashish.

Chromatography. Chemical method for detecting and identifying cannabinoids* present in unknown substances suspected of being marihuana. Substances are absorbed on a paper or column containing a solvent. Identity is determined by comparing movement with a known material.

Chronic. Long-term usage as opposed to acute.

Chuckers, chucks. Appetite, craving, hunger for food after smoking marihuana. *See* Blind Munchies.

Chunk. Hashish.

Churus. Marihuana. From *charas; see* appendix.

Cigar. Thick marihuana cigarette. *See also* Bomber.
1969: "A marihuana cigarette close to the size of a cigar." (Geller and Boas, *Drug Beat*, p. 71).

Citroli. Potent hashish from Nepal.

Clarabelle. THC—Tetrahydrocannabinol, the active ingredient in marihuana.

Clean. 1. To remove stems and seeds from crude marihuana. 2. Not using drugs. 3. Not having drugs in your possession.
1961: "After he got it cleaned he started rolling joints." (Hughes, *Fantastic Lodge*, p. 145).

Clime's on you. High*; intoxicated (1930s-1940s).

Clip. Device for holding butt (roach) of marihuana cigarette. *See* Bridge, Crutch, Jefferson Airplane.

Clipped. Arrested.

Club. Place for smoking marihuana.
1938: "Another who was particularly informative had been proprietor of a 'club,' 'den,' or 'tea-pad,' slang for places where reefer smokers congregate." (Yawger, "Marihuana," p. 355).

Club des Haschischins (Hashish Club). A social club of French writers and artists who met on a monthly basis in Paris's Latin Quarter at the Hotel Lauzun during the 1830s-1840s to fraternize and use hashish. Founded by Theophile Gautier, the club included such notables as Alexander Dumas, Victor Hugo, Charles Baudelaire, Gerard de Nerval, and Ferdinand Boissard.

Coasting. Feeling euphoric following drug use; under the influence of marihuana.

Cocktail. Marihuana butt placed into the end of a tobacco cigarette.
1968: ". . . 'cocktails' ['roaches'] twisted onto the end of a regular cigarette." (Goode, *Marihuana*, p. 8).
1969: "The 'cocktail' method—one of the most popular means of consuming roaches. . . ." (Geller and Boas, *Drug Beat*, p. 72).

Cola. Flowering tops of marihuana plant.

Coldwell, Samuel. Marihuana dealer. First person to be sentenced, along with Moses Baca, a marihuana user, under Marihuana Tax Act of 1937. Coldwell received a four-year prison term and a $1,000 fine; Baca, eighteen months. Sentenced in Denver, Colorado.

Collared. Arrested; *see also* Busted.

Colombian. Marihuana from Colombia; very potent. Comes in various colors, for example, gold, red.
1971: "It's Colombian smoke." (Woodley, *Dealer*, p. 127).
1974: "I had flown to Florida to arrange a score for some Colombian." (*High Times*, vol. 1, no. 1, p. 11).
1976: ". . . the best Colombian Gold we've ever seen." (*High Times*, November, p. 10).
1976: "The best so far has been a cross between Thai and Colombian Red." (*High Times*, November, p. 102).
1979: "Colombian Gold, which is offered at $15 a bag. . . ." (Goldman, *Grass Roots*, p. 27).

1980: One week you might have Colombian gold tops at sixty dollars
an ounce." (Novak, *High Culture*, p. 102).

Color. Acapulco Gold, Gold Colombian, Red Lebanese, and such. The
colors of marihuana originating from different countries. The colors
have nothing to do with potency but instead are due to loss of green-
colored chlorophyll. Absence of green color reveals the influence of
various resins contained in marihuana, each of which has a color of its
own. Colors also may be due to nutritional deficiencies experienced by
the plant, for example, red indicates phosphorus deficiency; yellow,
potassium deficiency. Color also may come from the material holding
the marihuana together, for example, honey, camel dung.

Columbus Black. Marihuana from Ohio; black in color.

Come down. 1. Return to normal condition after being high.* 2. Emotional depression after smoking marihuana.
1961: ". . . the coming down, which I don't dig on pot at all." (Hughes,
Fantastic Lodge, p. 74).

Come home. *See* Come down.

Commercial. Marihuana or hashish sold to buyers in contrast to
"black" marihuana or hashish used by dealers for their own enjoyment.
1971: ". . . the man who plants large fields of commercial dope,
doesn't take time to pinch back the plants." (Coyote Man, *Buzz*,
p. 3).
1976: "There was some dude who was raving about some of the hash
he'd smoked. All commercial stuff." (Sorfleet, "Dealing," p.
146).
1978: ". . . the kind that's known in the dealing trade simply—and often
contemptuously—as 'commercial'. . . ." (*High Times*, July, p. 38).

Committee on Cannabis Indica of the Ohio State Medical Society.
First (1860) formally organized committee in the United States to ex-
amine and discuss marihuana. Mainly concerned with therapeutic uses.

Con. To cheat, deceive. *See* Burned.

Conga. Marihuana from Africa.

Congo Brown. Potent marihuana from Africa; brown in color.

Congo Mataby. Potent marihuana from Africa.

Connect. Locate or buy marihuana or any drug.

Conncction. 1. Drug seller. 2. Obtain drugs.

1936: "Connection." (Maurer, "Argot," p. 120).
1966: "He searches for a 'connection.' " (*Village Voice*, December 1,
p. 20).

Contact High. 1. Intoxicated from breathing marihuana smoke exhaled
by others. 2. Euphoric state resulting from being where marihuana is
smoked without actually smoking it.
1968: "You don't have to get high, but you're going to be around
it . . . and people are going to be doing it, and you're going
to get contact high." (Gross, *Flower People*, p. 2).

Controlled Substance Act. Part of the Comprehensive Drug Abuse Prevention and Control Act (1970). This Act provided five categories
("Schedules") for psychoactive drugs, depending on their perceived
harmfulness, abuse potential, and accepted medical usage. Marihuana
is included under Schedule 1 along with heroin, which means it has
the highest potential for abuse, highest dependency liability, and no
currently accepted medical usage. Violation of the laws forbidding
manufacture, distribution, or disposal can result in a prison term of up
to fifteen years for a first offense and a fine of $5,000. For a second
offense, penalties include prison term of up to thirty years and a fine
of $50,000. Simple possession of marihuana was reduced to a mis-
demeanor.* Mandatory minumum sentences for users was abolished.
The law was signed in 1970 by President Nixon and went into effect
in May 1971. The law replaced previous drug laws concerning narcotics
and "dangerous drugs" such as Boggs, Harrison, and Marihuana Tax
Acts.

Cool. In control; aware; indifferent; aloof; smart; knowledgeable.

Cool it. Stop.

Cooler. Jail.

Cop. 1. Police officer. 2. To buy; steal; take. 3. To admit to something.
1968: " 'Copping' [buying] marihuana is, to a great number of smokers,
the most exciting event in which they can participate." (Rosevear,
Pot, p. 36).
1969: "When the pothead cops his purchase of marihuana, he prefers to
buy in large amounts." (Geller and Boas, *Drug Beat*, p. 68).

Cop a buy. Purchase marihuana.
1968: "The most common way of acquiring a 'stash' [private supply]
of marihuana is to 'cop' [buy] it." (Bloomquist, *Marihuana*,
p. 53).

Cop a match. To purchase a small amount of marihuana. *See* Matchbox.
1971: "Cop a match." (Folb, *Black Argot*, p. 8).

Cop a plea. To plead guilty to a lesser crime to receive a lighter sentence
rather than contesting a more serious charge and, if found guilty, receiving a harsher sentence.

Cop out. 1. To give up; to back out at the last minute. 2. To plead
guilty. 3. To stop using marihuana.

Coyote. Dishonest drug dealer.

Crash. 1. Unpleasant feeling coming out of drug experience. *See*
Come down. 2. To enter someone's home to stay for a short time.
3. To fall asleep after drug use.

Crash Pad. Place to stay during last phases of drug experience.

Crazy. 1. Under influence of marihuana (1940s). 2. Exceptional; excellent; good.
1946: "Let's knock ourselves crazy." (Charen and Perelman, "Marihuana Addicts," p. 678).
1955: *"I had a feeling I must go*
And blast some crazy pot. "
(Braddy, "Anonymous Verses," p. 130).

Creeper Joint. Place where marihuana smoker is robbed while he is
under the influence of the drug.
1938: "Creeper joint." (Berger, *New Yorker*, March 12, p. 47).
1952: "Let's get out of here, Lukey, it's a creep joint." (Mandell,
Flee the Angry Strangers, p. 132).

Crowley, Aleister (1875-1947). Called the "Great Beast" by his followers. Crowley was an early advocate of psychoactive drug use. He is
also the author of *The Psychology of Hashish:*

> 'Perhaps hashish is the drug which "loosens the girders of the soul," but is
> in itself neither good nor bad. Perhaps, as Baudelaire thinks, it merely ex-
> aggerates and distorts the natural man and his mood of the moment.' The
> whole of Ludlow's wonderful introspection seems to me to fortify this
> suggestion.

> Well, then, let me see whether by first exalting myself mystically and con-
> tinuing my invocations while the drug dissolved the matrix of the diamond
> Soul, that diamond might not manifest limpid and sparkling, a radiance
> 'not of the Sun, nor of the Moon, nor of the Stars'; and then, of course, I

remembered that this ceremonial intoxication constitutes the supreme ritual
of all religions. (*The Psychology of Hashish*, pp. 100-101).

Crutch. Device to hold marihuana cigarette butt [roach*] so that it
won't burn the fingers.
1938: ". . . experienced smokers who sometimes hold the cigarette in
the split end of a match. . . . Such a holder in the New Orleans
vernacular is known as a 'crutch.' " (Walton, *Marihuana*, p. 48).
1944: "When it gets to be very short, a split match called a 'crutch' is
used to hold the 'roach.' " (*Shock Magazine*, reprinted in Silver
and Aldrich, *Dope Chronicles*, p. 279).

Cube. Gram of hashish.

Cucaracha, La. Battle hymn of the Mexican revolution under Pancho
Villa, following his capture of the town of Torreon in Mexico. Later
La Cucaracha became a popular American musical hit. The song is
about the cockroach's inability to walk without marihuana.

Culiacan. Potent marihuana from Mexico.

Cured. Marihuana soaked in sugar water and then dried. Purpose is to
increase its weight. *See* Sugared.
1972: "One of the constant issues of conversation for both street buyers and street dealers considering the purchase of a key is whether
the marihuana has been 'cured in sugar'—a process which results
in increasing the weight but not the 'high.' " (Cavan, *Hippies*, p.
127).

Cut. To dilute marihuana with another substance like oregano or catnip
to increase its bulk.
1965: "He admits he could profit by 'cutting' his marihuana with
oregano." (Goldstein, "College Scene," p. 214).
1967: "Our job is to cut it and clean it and package it for sale." (Ric,
Esquire, September, p. 190).

Cut off. Insensible from use of too much drug.
1955: "I'm cut off from all of you." (Braddy, "Anonymous Verses,"
p. 132).

Cut out. To leave.

Cysolithic Hairs. Hairlike structures on the surface of the marihuana
leaf that arch over the resin-producing trichome glands and storage
sessile glands and protect them from direct sunlight.

D

Dagga. Marihuana.
1955: "Dagga." (Braddy, "Narcotic Argot," p. 87).
1970: "A few dagga smokers were booked in Los Angeles." (*Current Slang*, vol. 4, p. 4).

DaOrta, Garcia (1501-1568). Spanish physician who served in Portuguese India. DaOrta wrote about effects of marihuana and other drugs in *Colloquies on the Simples and Drugs of India* (1563). This book became the most influential text on drugs in the West for several centuries and the primary source on marihuana's effects until the eighteenth century.

Dawamesc. Favorite hashish confection of members of Club des Haschischins*; *see* appendix.

DEA. Drug Enforcement Administration. Created in 1973 by President Nixon by merging BNDD* and ODALE.* Currently the main federal agency concerned with enforcement of drug laws.

Dealer. Supplier of marihuana. A dealer is often distinguished from a pusher* in that a dealer sells "soft" drugs like marihuana, whereas a pusher sells "hard" drugs like heroin.
1938: "When his stock runs low he calls a dealer at 110th Street and Lennox Avenue and an automobile brings a fresh supply." (Berger, *New Yorker*, March 12, p. 48).
1965: "He said he wanted to start dealing pot." (Brown, *Manchild*, p. 161).
1966: "Dealers vary in the ways they regard the threat of being busted." (*Village Voice*, December 1, p. 21).
1971: "Dealers meant just about anyone who could get up enough cash to buy dope in quantity, sell it off at a profit, and then buy more." (Hall, *Heads*, p. 19).

Dealing. Selling marihuana.

Deadwood. Undercover police officer posing as drug user.

Debris. Marihuana particles, for example, seeds, stems, left after cleaning. *See* clean.

Deck. Pack of marihuana cigarettes.
1943: "Deck." (*Time*, July 19, p. 54).
1959: "Deck." (Schmidt, *Narcotics*, p. 38).

Decriminalization. Reduction of penalties for possession of small amounts of marihuana. Currently, the following states have decriminalized marihuana possession: Alaska, California, Colorado, Maine, Minnesota, Mississippi, Nebraska, New York, North Carolina, Ohio, and Oregon.

The penalty for possession of up to one ounce in most of these states is a fine of $0 to $250. Maine has no restrictions on amount in possession. Alaska allows any amount for possession as long as it is for private, personal use. Arizona, Missouri, and Montana, on the other hand, have prison sentences of up to life for possession of these same amounts.

Delirium. Temporary state of mental disturbance with confusion, incoherence, or hallucinations. Sometimes associated with use of high doses of marihuana.

Delta-9-tetrahydrocannabinol (Δ^9-THC, THC). Principle active constituent in marihuana responsible for its psychoactive properties. THC was first isolated in 1964 in Israel. (*See* Cannabinoids.) The amount of THC contained in plant depends on plant strain, climate, soil conditions, and method of harvesting. Different parts of the marihuana plant contain different amounts of THC. Generally, the higher the plant from the ground, the greater the THC content on its parts.

Delusion. A false belief.

Dependence. A condition occurring as a result of continuous use of certain drugs. Dependence can be either physical, psychological, or both. Physical dependence (addiction) is an adaptation of the body to the presence of a drug, such that its absence precipitates a withdrawal syndrome. (*See also* Addiction.) Psychological dependence is a condition in which the user feels a desire, but not a compulsion to continue drug use for a sense of well-being and feels discomfort when deprived of it. There is little tendency to increase the dosage. Marihuana does not cause physical dependence but may result in psychological dependence in certain individuals.

Depersonalization. Loss of sense of "self."

Depressant. A drug that reduces activity of bodily organs, especially the brain; for example, alcohol, barbiturates, tranquilizers.

Destroyed. Physically or psychologically exhausted; unable to cope. *See also* Wasted.

Deuce Bag. Two dollars' worth of marihuana.

Deuce someone. Sell someone two marihuana cigarettes.
1938: " 'Deuce me, man,' he said." (Berger, *New Yorker*, March 12,
    p. 48).

Devine, Reverend Robert James. Barnstorming crusader against marihuana in Michigan during the 1930s. Authored two antimarihuana
books, *The Menace of Marihuana* and *The Moloch of Marihuana*.

Dew Rot (or ret). Exposing dry hemp stalks to the weather so that they
will rot and fibers can be peeled from stalk.

Dibenzopyran System. Chemical notation for describing cannabinoids.
Formal name for active cannabinoid in marihuana according to this
system is delta-9-THC. Another chemical system, monoterpenoid,
refers to this same compound as delta-1-THC.

Dig. Understand.

Dime Bag. Ten dollars' worth of marihuana.
1967: "Kids chip in $5 and $10 (for nickel and dime bags)." (*Look*,
    August 18, p. 12).
1967: "Never buy pot from the petty dealer of 'nickel and dime bags.' "
    (*Newsweek*, July 24, p. 47).

Ding. Marihuana.

Dinky Dow. Marihuana cigarette. Term used by American soldiers in
Vietnam.
1968: "Dinky dow conk out: Marihuana cigarette." (*Marihuana Review*,
    vol. 1, no. 1, p. 4).

Dioecious. Botanical term referring to plants like marihuana that contain only male staminate or female pistillate flowers on each plant in
contrast to monoecious plants, which contain both male and female
parts on the same plant.

Dirt Grass. Low-potency marihuana.

Dirty. 1. Uncleaned marihuana; contains seeds, stems, and leaves.
2. Possessing marihuana or any other drug.
1972: "Yesterday I was dirty, but today I had nothing." (Hall, *Heads*,
    p. 55).
Do. To take marihuana or any other drug.
1961: "I was doing up six and ten joints a day." (Hughes, *Fantastic
    Lodge*, p. 74).
1972: "Don't get so uptight about me; I haven't been doing that many
    drugs." (Hall, *Heads*, p. 15).

Do a joint. Smoke marihuana.

Do up. Smoke marihuana.
1967: "Let's do up the joint." (Shorris, *Ofay*, p. 65).
1971: "Dave had several grams of hash, which we planned to do up on the slopes." (Hall, *Heads*, p. 21).
1977: "Do up." (Lentini, *Vice*, p. 135).

Doing your business. Smoking marihuana.

Dona Juanita. Marihuana.
1955: "Dona Juanita." (Braddy, "Narcotic Argot," p. 83).

Doobie, Dubbe, Dubee, Dubie, Duby. Marihuana.
1968: "Dubie." (U. California, *Folklore*, p. 418).
1971: "Duby." (Landy, *Underground Dictionary*, p. 72).
1972: "Dubie." (Smith and Gray, *It's So Good*, p. 201).
1977: "Dubbe." (Lentini, *Vice*, p. 135).
1978: "I settled onto bed and started to roll a nice doobie." *(High Times*, July, p. 15).

Dope. Any drug. Most popular term for marihuana in 1970s.
1928: ". . . hashish, the dope so common in India." (*Chicago Tribune*, July 1, p. 12).
1934: "I didn't know it was dope." (De Lenoir, *Hundredth Man*, p. 226).
1957: "I saw many other dope 'tea pads' (marijuana dens)." (Danforth and Horan, *Big City*, p. 126).
1979: "He's handing out a lot of good dope for free." (Goldman, *Grass Roots*, p. 23).

Dope Den. Place where marihuana or other drugs are used.
1965: "Enter a dope den, and quote enigmatic Scripture to reefer-smoking delinquents." (Himes, *Imabelle*, p. 33).

Dope Head. Regular marihuana user. *See also* Pot Head.

Dope Lawyer. Attorney who specializes in defending persons accused of violation of drug laws.
1976: "How did you get started as a dope lawyer?" (*High Times*, September, p. 23).

Dope Pipe. Pipe for smoking marihuana or hashish.
1970: "You could reach a dope pipe or a Polaroid camera standing anywhere in the pad." (Sanders, *Shards*, p. 21).

Dope Smoke. Marihuana; hashish.
1961: "Dope smoke." (Partridge, *Dictionary*, p. 199).

Doped Cigarettes. Marihuana.
1939: "Doped cigarettes." (DeLeeuw, *Flower*, p. 229).
1949: ". . . doped cigarettes." (Chandler, *Little Sister*, p. 271).

Doper. Marihuana user; any frequent user of psychoactive drugs.

Dopester. *See* Doper.

Doubleheader. Two marihuana cigarettes smoked at the same time.
Purpose is to increase amount of smoke breathed in.
1970: "Doubleheader." (Brennan, *Drugs*, p. 65).
1973: "Doubleheader." (Maurer, *Narcotics*, p. 403).

Down. 1. Unpleasant aftereffects of smoking marihuana. 2. Return to
normal state following marihuana use.
1944: "A cold shower will also have the effect of bringing the person
'down.' " (*La Guardia Report*, p. 13).

Drag. 1. Deep inhalation of tobacco or marihuana cigarette. 2. Boring,
unpleasant situation.
1938: "They took long violent drags, seeming to swallow the smoke
and inhale it simultaneously." (Rowell, *David Dare*, p. 6).
1955: "To drag on this thing was like leaning over a chimney and inhaling." (Kerouac, *Road*, p. 283).
1956: "He kept dragging at the reefer." (Hunter, *Second Ending*, p.
248).
1960: "Joyce took two more drags on the stick." (De Mexico, *Marijuana Girl*, p. 46).
1972: "Irmy sighed and took a slow drag on the joint." (Woodley,
Dealer, p. 50).

Dragged. State of anxiety after smoking marihuana some time previously.
1965: "She's dragged because she's high like that." (Becker, *Outsiders*,
p. 56).

Dream Stick. Marihuana cigarette.
1959: "Dream stick." (Schmidt, *Narcotics*, p. 45).

Dress. To clear appending matter from hemp fiber. The equivalent of
cleaning for marihuana. *See* clean.

Drink Texas Tea. Smoke marihuana.
1959: "Drink Texas Tea: To smoke hashishi cigarettes." (Schmidt,
Narcotics, p. 46).

Drop a joint. To smoke a marihuana cigarette.

Drop out. To detach oneself from everyday concerns.

Drug. Although thought of usually as any substance used to treat disease, a more proper definition is any substance that affects bodily function, including any material—plant, powder, fluid, solid, or gas—that can be eaten, drunk, injected, sniffed, inhaled, or absorbed from the skin.

Drunk. Intoxicated on marihuana.

1938: "A viper can get drunk on anywhere from one to four or five cigarettes—ten to fifty cents' worth—while it would cost him a dollar or two for a whiskey jag." (Berger, *New Yorker*, March 12, p. 50).

1938: "Marihuana is not a habit-former like opium and cocaine. From a so-called 'drunk,' there are no hangover symptoms and there are no known fatalities." (Yawger, "Marihuana," p. 357).

Dubbe, Dubee, Dubie, Duby. *See* Doobie.

Duck. Coarse hemp cloth used for sails, tents, and other sturdy materials.

Duke in. To expose an undercover police officer.

Dumas, Alexander (1802-1870). French writer and member of the Club des Haschischins.* Best known for his tales of adventure, including *The Count of Monte Cristo*, which uses hashish as a plot device in one chapter.

Duquenois Test. Forensic test used to detect presence of marihuana. The test substance is mixed with vanillin, acetaldehyde, alcohol, and hydrochloric acid. If marihuana is present, the mixture turns violet.

Dust. 1. Marihuana cigarette to which heroin or opium has been added. *See also* A(tom) Bomb, Candy a J. 2. Hashish.

Dynamite. Potent marihuana; extraordinarily good; superlative. Originally used in reference to narcotics.

1951: "At Boys High School, according to the agent, 'John' overheard a group of boys in the toilet talking about the 'dynamite' they had smoked the previous night." (*New York Times*, June 14, p. 22/2).

1952: "I got some dynamite, it's from India." (Mandell, *Flee the Angry Strangers*, p. 162).

1962: "Dynamite." (Wentworth and Flexner, *Dictionary*, p. 161).

1970: "That's dynamite grass." (Goode, *Marihuana Smokers*, p. 327).

Dynamiters. Potent marihuana cigarettes.

1959: "Dynamiters." (Murtagh and Harris, *Who Live in Shadows*, p. 201).

E

Elbow. A pound of marihuana.
1976: "That stuff in the drawer is an elbow of Columbian [*sic*]."
(U. California, *Folklore*, p. 76).

Electric Butter. Marihuana sauteed in butter.
1970: "Electric butter." (Brennan, *Drugs*, p. 67).

El Paso Ordinance. First (June 24, 1914) local ordinance passed in an American city outlawing sale, barter, exchange, or possession of marihuana within its jurisdiction. Penalty for violation was $50 fine or three months in jail.

Euphoria. State of happiness, pleasure, contentment. Main reason for using marihuana is to achieve this state.

Euphoriant. Drug causing euphoria.*

Extractum cannabis. Extract of marihuana. First listed in the U.S. Pharmacopoeia in 1850. Continued to be included in the Pharmacopoeia until 1942.

E-Z Wider. First (1972) specially designed rolling paper for making marihuana cigarettes. These papers are wider than traditional cigarette papers.
1979: ". . . rolling joints with oversize papers called e-z widers." (Goldman, *Grass Roots*, p. 23).

F

Faggot. Marihuana.
1959: "Faggot." (Schmidt, *Narcotics*, p. 58).

Fake a blast. Pretend to inhale marihuana cigarette or pretend to become high.*
1968: "Fake a blast." (Wolfe, *Hippies*, p. 204).

Fall out. Fall asleep after smoking marihuana.

Far out. Excellent; superior; unusual; remarkable; sensational.

Farmer. A nondrug user; someone naive; a square.*

Fat. 1. Thick. 2. Possessing a large amount of marihuana.
1972: "Some believe in 'fat' or 'moderately fat' joints as minimally

adequate for the aim of two or more people getting high."
(Cavan, *Hippies*, p. 127).

1977: "I would have had to pay from $25 (asking price) to $18 (selling price) for a fat lid." (*High Times*, January, p. 9).

Fat Jay. Thick marihuana cigarette, thickened because of low-potency.

Fatty. Thick marihuana cigarette. *See also* Bomber, Fat Jay.

Fay Hound. Homosexual marihuana user.

1946: "Fay hound." (Charen and Perelman, "Marihuana Addicts," p. 678).

Fed. Federal narcotics agent.

1955: "The Feds got me busted for one little sale." (Braddy, "Anonymous Verses," p. 133).

Federal Beef. Federal narcotics offense.

Federal Bureau of Narcotics. First (1930) federal agency specifically organized to control illicit drugs. The Federal Bureau of Narcotics was initially responsible for enforcement of the Harrison Narcotic Act (1915). Powers were based on federal taxing powers and therefore the agency was part of treasury department. After 1937, the bureau also became responsible for federal enforcement of the Marihuana Tax Act. The bureau was abolished in 1968 and replaced by the Bureau of Drug Abuse Control, which also was abolished and replaced by the Bureau of Narcotics and Dangerous Drugs (BNDD). The BNDD was removed from the treasury department and made part of the justice department.

Feel like the world's against me. Suffering from lack of marihuana.
1938: "Feel like the world's against me." (Walton, *Marihuana*, p. 195).

Felony. Any offense for which a sentence is to be served in a state or federal prison. Each state has its own definition, based on maximum sentence.

Fennel. Marihuana.
1970: "It was cannabis, hemp, weed, gage, fennel, all these names." (Sanders, *Shards*, p. 52).

Fiend. Drug addict; someone who cannot control his drug usage.
1917: "A 'marihuana fiend' is a source of real danger." (Smith, Department of Agriculture, p. 7).

Fine Stuff. Finely manicured marihuana.
1955: "Fine stuff." (Braddy, "Narcotic Argot," p. 87).

Finger. Quantity of hashish about the size and shape of a finger.
1979: "Often all they get is crudely made hashish, which looks like the
fingers most of us know." (Cherniak, *Hashish*, p. 137).

Finger, To. To inform.

Fink. Informer; betrayer.

Fink, To. To inform.

Fire up. To light a marihuana cigarette; to smoke marihuana or hashish.
1960: "Beats gather in a desert to fire up some marihuana." (Chiardi,
Saturday Review, p. 12).
1973: "Fire up." (Maurer, *Narcotics*, p. 406).

Flag. Arrest. *See* Bust, Busted.
1971: "They flagged my reefer man yesterday." (Woodley, *Dealer*,
p. 86).

Flake. To fall asleep from taking too much marihuana.
1972: "Flake." (Folb, *Black Argot*, p. 90).

Flip, Flip Out, Flipped. To have an unpleasant experience following
marihuana use, or, conversely, to have an enjoyable reaction.
1965: "I was so high, and I got real flipped." (Becker, *Outsiders*, p. 57).
1969: "Flip out." (Geller and Boas, *Drug Beat*, p. xvii).

Floating. Lightheadedness from smoking marihuana.
1936: "Floating." (Maurer, "Argot of Underworld," p. 121).
1937: "The girl was 'floating' now, a term given to marihuana intoxication." (Anslinger, *American Magazine*, p. 19).
1937: "There is no girl who can find the strength to resist once she
has begun 'to float.'" (Cooper, *Here's to Crime*, p. 335).
1943: "The smoker is then said to be 'high' or 'floating.'" (*Time*,
July 19, p. 54).

Flying. Lightheadedness from smoking marihuana.
1938: "Flying." (Walton, *Marihuana*, p. 195).
1952: "Flying." (Lannoy and Masterson, "Hophead Jargon," p. 25).
1969: "Flying." (Geller and Boas, *Drug Beat*, p. xviii).

Foxy. Intuitive feeling from smoking marihuana.
1938: "Foxy." (Walton, *Marihuana*, p. 195).

Fraho, Frajo. Marihuana cigarette.
1952: "Frajo." (Lannoy and Masterson, "Hophead Jargon," p. 25).
1970: "Frajo." (Cromwell, *Slang*, p. 76).

Freak. Habitual heavy user of drugs; user obsessed with marihuana or any other drug.
1967: "Freak." (Brown, *Hippies*, p. 218).
1968: "Freak." (Wolfe, *Hippies*, p. 204).
1969: "Freak." (Geller and Boas, *Drug Beat*, p. xviii).

Freak out. To hallucinate; become stuporous; to have an unpleasant drug reaction.
1967: "Freak out." (Brown, *Hippies*, p. 218).
1968: "Most of the real heads were completely freaked out." (*New York Times*, January 11, p. 18/7).
1971: I got really high; in fact, I nearly freaked out." (Hall, *Heads*, p. 12).

Free Grass, Free Smoke. Marihuana remaining after most has been sold. Kept for dealer's own use.
1968: "We'd come out with free grass." (Ric, *Esquire*, September, p. 101).
1976: "The occasional dealer, who deals only for 'free smoke' . . ." (Sorfleet, "Dealing," p. 130).

Freeze. To refuse to sell drugs.
1966: "I'm sick and he's put the freeze on." (Sutter, "Righteous Dope Fiend," p. 203).

Fried. Very high.*

Front, Front Cash, Fronting. 1. Selling marihuana on credit to another dealer. 2. To give payment before marihuana has been received.
1966: ". . . people who have been arrested before, may live as recluses, having a few trusted assistants to whom they 'front' drugs to sell for a commission." (*Village Voice*, December 1, p. 21).
1968: "There are three basic rules in dealing: Don't front money; test all drugs before you buy; and don't front money!" (Carey, *College Drug Scene*, p. 82).
1976: "I was dealing ten thousand dollars' worth of hash every three days, but it was all fronted." (Sorfleet, "Dealing," p. 133).
1980: "I supply other dealers, usually on a fronting basis." (Novak, *High Culture*, p. 111).

Fu. Marihuana (1930s-1940s).
1936: "The drug and cigarettes containing it are known as 'fu.' " (Spencer, "Marihuana," p. 300).
1937: ". . . it now is being called 'fu.' " (Cooper, *Here's to Crime*, p. 333).
1942: "Fu." (Berrey and Bark, *Thesaurus*, p. 474).

Fu Manchu. Marihuana smoker.
1959: "Fu manchu." (Schmidt, *Narcotics*, p. 64).

Full Blast. Very high.*
1967: "My high was on full blast." (Thomas, *Mean Streets*, p. 221).

Full Moon. Round cake of hashish.

Funny Cigarettes. Marihuana.
1949: "Funny cigarettes ain't all that one pushes." (Algren, *Man with the Golden Arm*, p. 30).

Funny Stuff. Marihuana.

Fuzz. Police.
1952: "I hate Fuzz worse'n poison." (Mandell, *Flee the Angry Strangers*, p. 231).
1966: "Fuzz, man, they want to bust you, they bust you, doesn't matter what the charge, that's the whole fuzz syndrome right there." (Farina, *Been Down So Long*, p. 64).

⎯⎯ G ⎯⎯⎯⎯⎯⎯⎯⎯⎯⎯⎯⎯⎯⎯⎯⎯⎯⎯⎯⎯

G-Man. Federal narcotics agent.
1945: "The G Man Got the T Man." Song recorded by C. P. Johnson.

Gage, Gauge, Guage. Marihuana. From *ganja*,* the term for marihuana in India and Jamaica; *see* appendix.
1946: "I was standing on The Corner pushing gauge." (Mezzrow and Wolfe, *Really the Blues*, p. 211).
1952: ". . . nursing Louella along to her first gauge high." (Mandell, *Flee the Angry Strangers*, p. 241).
1955: "You can carry about five sticks of gauge in the beard." (Witmore, *Solo*, p. 41).
1960: "Ain't nothing wrong with gauge." (De Mexico, *Marijuana Girl*, p. 119).
1965: "Three teen-age boys had a fifteen-year-old girl inside, all blowing gage." (Himes, *Imabelle*, p. 33).
1980: ". . . when you've picked up some gauge . . ." (Novak, *High Culture*, p. 115).

Gage, Gauge, Guage Butt. Marihuana cigarette.

Gage, Gauge, Guage Party. Gathering to smoke marihuana.
1946: "Gage party." (Charen and Perelman, "Marihuana Addicts," p. 678).

Gage in the Rough. Uncleaned marihuana.

Gainesville Green. Domestically grown marihuana from Florida.

Gallows Grass. Hemp.

Gang. Quantity of marihuana.
1944: "I should be sitting in the stables listening to the Hawk with a gang of hemp in my lap." (Marcovitz and Myers, "Marihuana Addict," p. 391).

Gangster. Marihuana.
1960. "Just go on and smoke that gangster." (Cooper, *Scene*, p. 308).
1969: "He was sucking a stick of gangster." (Iceberg Slim, *Pimp*, pp. 96-97).

Ganja. Marihuana.

Garbage. Low-potency marihuana.
1962: "They took several puffs and presently Howie said, 'Garbage.' " (Pritchie, *Savage Kick*, p. 26).

Gas. 1. Good time; pleasing, amusing incident. 2. Nitrous oxide.

Gash. Marihuana.
1968: "Gash." (Lindesmith, *Addict*, p. 251).

Gasper. Marihuana cigarette.
1960: "Gasper." (Wentworth and Flexner, *Dictionary*, p. 209).

Gates. Marihuana.
1968: "These terms will probably go out of style, as have the slightly outdated and rarely used words . . . gates . . ." (Goode, *Marihuana*, p. 3).
1969: "Cigarettes containing marihuana are home-made and are referred to as . . . 'gates' . . ." (Farnsworth, "Cannabis Sativa," p. 41).

Gauged. Intoxicated on marihuana; high.*
1957: " 'We'll get you real gauged tonight,' he said." (Danforth and Horan, *Big City*, p. 124).

Gautier, Pierre Jules Theophile (1811-1872). French writer. Gautier became interested in hashish through his acquaintance with Dr. J.

Moreau and subsequently founded the Club des Haschischins.* He was
one of the first European writers to describe the hashish experience
and thereby to acquaint others with its effects.

> "My body seemed to dissolve and I became transparent. Within my breast
> I perceived the hashish I had eaten in the form of an emerald scintillating
> with a million points of fire. My eyelashes elongated indefinitely, unrolling
> themselves like threads of gold on ivory spindles which spun of their own
> accord with dazzling rapidity. Around me poured streams of gems of every
> color, in ever-changing patterns like the play within a kaleidoscope. My com-
> rades appeared to me to be disfigured, part men, part plants. . . . So strange
> did they seem that I writhed with laughter. . . . My hearing became pro-
> digiously acute. I actually listened to the sound of colors. . . . Never has
> greater beauty immersed me in its flood." (Gautier, "Club des Haschischins,"
> trans. by Laurie, *Drugs*, p. 86).

Gazer. Federal narcotics officer.
1952: "Gazer." (Oursler and Smith, *Hooked*, p. 189).

Gear. Marihuana.
1954: "Those who deal in them on street corners, or cheap cafes, in
   worse dance halls and amusement arcades, may call them 'dope,'
   or 'kif,' or 'charge,' or 'gear,' or 'tea.' " (Bevan, *Everybody's*,
   June 12, p. 11).

Get down. Various meanings including smoking marihuana.
1972: "Get down." (Folb, *Black Argot*, p. 139).

Get it on. Various meanings including smoking marihuana.
1972: "Get it on." (Folb, *Black Argot*, p. 139).

Get off. Various meanings including becoming intoxicated from
smoking marihuana.
1977: "It takes a huge joint to get one person off." (*High Times*,
   January, p. 9).

Get on. Various meanings including smoking marihuana.

Giggle Smoke. Marihuana.
1937: "They are spoken of as . . . 'giggle smokes.' " (Anon., "Marihuana," p. 184).
1943: "Cigarettes made from it are . . . 'giggle smokes.' " (*Time*,
   July 19, p. 54).
1959: "Giggle smoke." (Schmidt, *Narcotics*, p. 68).
1968: "These terms will probably go out of style, as have the slightly

outdated and rarely used words . . . 'giggle-smoke' . . ." (Goode, *Marihuana*, p. 3).

Giggle Weed. Marihuana.
1951: "Before that, it was marijuana, which we call 'giggle weed.' "
(San Diego Evening Tribune, June 28, p. A1/4).

Go loco. Smoke marihuana. *See also* Loco Weed.
1961: "Go loco." (Partridge, *Dictionary*, p. 294).

Go straight. Give up marihuana or any other drug.

Gold. 1. Potent marihuana, for example, Acapulco Gold, Colombian Gold, Kona Gold.
1980: "I'm religiously smoking some delicious gold right now." (Novak, *High Culture*, p. 254).

Gold Leaf. 1. Potent marihuana. 2. Acapulco Gold.* 3. Marihuana originating from a foreign country.
1925: "Gold Leaf Strut." Song recorded by Original New Orleans Rhythm Kings.
1946: "Man, this is some golden-leaf I brought up from New Orleans." (Mezzrow and Wolfe, *Really the Blues*, p. 60).
1961: "He earned as he went, by judicious minor transactions in the golden leaf." (Russell, *Sound*, p. 86).

Gold Leaf Special. Potent marihuana cigarette. *See* Gold Leaf, Special.

Gonga Smudge. Marihuana cigarette.
1939: "Gonga smudge." (Pollock, *Underworld Speaks*, p. 20).

Goober. Marihuana cigarette.

Good Time Man. Drug seller.
1971: "Good time man." (Eschholz and Rosa, "Slang," p. 12).

Goof. Marihuana user.
1952: "Goof." (Oursler and Smith, *Hooked*, p. 189).

Goof Balls. Marihuana.
1968: "Goof balls: '. . . pills made up of cannabis resin.' " (Dawtry, *Drug Abuse*, p. 90).

Goof Butt. Marihuana cigarette.
1938: "Marihuana cigarettes have a dozen names. Right now they are 'sticks,' 'reefers,' 'Mary Anns,' 'tea,' 'gyves,' 'guage'—or 'goofy butts.' " (Berger, *New Yorker*, March 12, p. 47).

1939: " 'Reefers,' or 'goof-butts' as the marijuana cigarettes are called." (Sullivan, *Double Life*, p. 226).
1943: "They blast the goof butt." (*Time*, July 19, p. 54).
1952: "Goof butt." (Lannoy and Masterson, "Hophead Jargon," p. 26).
1959: "Goof butt." (Schmidt, *Narcotics*, p. 71).

Goofed (up). Intoxicated on marihuana, barbiturates, or opium.
1955: "Yeah, one good drag and you're goofed to the sky." (Ellson, *Rock*, p. 36).
1957: "Vinnie was digging the conversation but was goofed with the tea and didn't bother to say anything." (Selby, *Last Exit*, p. 40).
1958: "I goofed and just wanted / To be left alone." (Braddy, "Anonymous Verses," p. 136).

Goofing. 1. Smoking marihuana. 2. Teasing one who is high on marihuana.

Gouger. Marihuana smoker.
1959: "Gouger." (Schmidt, *Narcotics*, p. 70).

Gow. Marihuana cigarette. Originally any narcotic.

Gowster. Marihuana user. Originally a narcotics user.
1960: "Gowster." (Wentworth and Flexner, *Dictionary*, p. 226).

Grass. Marihuana. The most popular term for marihuana in the 1960s, although term originated much earlier.
1943: "Marihuana may be called grass." (*Time*, July 19, p. 54).
1952: "Grass." (Lannoy and Masterson, "Hophead Jargon," p. 26).
1955: "I don't want no sweet grass to smoke." (Ellson, *Rock*, p. 46).
1966: " 'Grass,' said Mojo. 'Mexican Brown. Very clean quality I can assure you.' " (Farina, *Been Down So Long*, p. 26).
1966: "The dealer shows his money and the connection brings out the grass." (*Village Voice*, December 1, p. 3).
1967: *I Couldn't Smoke the Grass on My Father's Lawn*. Title of book by M. Chaplin.

Grass Action. Buying or selling marihuana.

Grass Brownies. Cookies baked with marihuana. *See* Alice B. Toklas.
1977: "Grass brownies." (Lentini, *Vice*, p. 137).

Grass Eater. Marihuana user.
1959: "Grass eater." (Schmidt, *Narcotics*, p. 72).

Grass Party. Gathering to smoke marihuana.

1946: "Grass party." (Charen and Perelman, "Marihuana Addicts," p. 678).

Grass Pipe. Pipe for smoking marihuana or hashish.
1968: ". . . grass pipes." (*New York Times*, January 11, p. 18/1).

Grasshopper. 1. Marihuana user. 2. Luggage for smuggling marihuana.
1948: "Grasshopper." (Gottschalk and Cowdry, *Language*, p. 6).
1968: "Grasshopper." (Lindesmith, *Addict*, p. 257).
1970: "Grasshopper." (Gomerly, *Drugs*, p. 183).
1976: "They come on slick as a whistle, pulled guns, tied us up, and ran off with two full grasshoppers." (*High Times*, November, p. 96).

Greefa, Greefo, Grefa, Greta, Griefo, Grifa, Griffa, Grifo. Marihuana.
1933: "The Mexican beet-field workers have introduced a new problem—the smoking in cigarettes and pipes, of marihuana or grifo." (Hayes and Bowery, "Marihuana," p. 1091).
1936: "Greefo." (Maurer, "Argot of Underworld," p. 121).
1938: "The drug is known by many different names such as . . . 'greefo' . . . " (Yawger, "Marihuana," p. 351).
1942: "Griffa." (Berrey and Bark, *Thesaurus*, p. 474).
1956: "The Negro hornman or drummer is often on . . . grefa." (Longstreet, *Real Jazz*, p. 144).

Green. 1. New marihuana smoker. 2. Marihuana.
1938: "Green." (Walton, *Marihuana*, p. 195).
1976: "F. Would like a quarter-pound of that Green I got from you the other day." (Sorfleet, "Dealing," p. 131).

Green Griff. Marihuana.

Green Moroccan. Hashish from Morocco; green in color.

Griefer. Marihuana smoker.
1961: "Griefer." (Partridge, *Dictionary*, p. 307).

Grifado. Intoxicated on marihuana or other drugs.
1970: "Grifado." (*Current Slang*, vol. 5, no. 3, p. 7).

Gungeon, Gunja, Gunjeh. 1. Marihuana. 2. Marihuana from Jamaica.
3. Term for most potent form of marihuana during 1940s, which sold for one dollar per cigarette. *See also* Black Gungeon.
1888: ". . . a dry green shrub, which I subsequently learned was gunjeh (the dried tops and leaves of the hemp plant), for smoking." (Anon., "Hashish House in New York," p. 181).

1944: " 'Gungeon' is considered by the marihuana smoker as the highest grade of marihuana." (*La Guardia Report*, p. 9).

Gunny. Marihuana.

Guru. Guide or authority; one who initiates someone else into drug use.

Gyves. Marihuana cigarettes. Possibly mistaken for "jives."
1938: "Gyves." (Berger, *New Yorker*, March 12, p. 47).

H

Habituation. *See* Dependence.

Hackel. Steel-toothed comb for removing debris from hemp fiber.

Had. To be taken advantage of.

Haidar (Haydar). Persian founder of religious order of Sufis. Haidar is said to have discovered hashish in A.D. 1155 and introduced it to his followers, hence the close association between hashish and the Sufi religion.

Haidar, Cup of. Hashish.

Haidar, Emerald Cup of. Hashish.

Hallucinogen. From the Greek word, *halucinari*—to wander mentally. A substance producing hallucinations, that is, perceptions unrelated to external stimuli, for example, LSD, mescaline, peyote, psilocybin. Marihuana also is considered in this category but is not as characteristic.

Hang in. Keep trying.

Hang loose. Relax; be calm; be cool.

Hangout. Place to gather, associate, congregate with others of similar temperament and interests.

Hang-up. A bother, concern.

Happening. Any event.

Happy Cigarette. Marihuana.

Harrison Act (Public Law No. 233). U.S. antinarcotics law. The Harrison Act came into effect March 1, 1915. It required dealers in narcotics to register with the Bureau of Internal Revenue and pay a small fee for a tax stamp. Narcotics users were not permitted to receive these stamps. Marihuana was not included in the law, but the tax-stamp method of regulation became the basis for later federal antimarihuana legislation.

Hash Cannon. Apparatus for smoking marihuana or hashish. Same as carburetor.*
1970: "Hash cannon." (Brennan, *Drugs*, p. 70).

Hash Oil. Distillate of marihuana or hashish. Viscous and very potent. Marihuana is extracted in boiling alcohol, which dissolves cannabinoids. Noncannabinoids are strained off. The solvent is then evaporated, leaving concentrated oil containing 40 to 60 percent THC. Appeared in United States during 1971. *See* One, Son of One.
1976: " 'Hash oil' is estimated to be ten times as potent as hashish." (Sorfleet, "Dealing," p. 128).
1977: "Hash oil never made it from the gourmet shop to the super-market." (*High Times*, February, p. 68).
1978: "The most potent form of THC comes in hash oil." (*Playboy*, September, p. 220).

Hashasheen. Loud, unruly people (Arabic). A term of reproach. The plural of hashash and possibly the origin of the English word "assassin." Assassins* were terrorists who allegedly used hashish. However, the origin of the word probably came about as a result of their being called hashasheen—unruly—a pun on the hashish eater; through the centuries, the pun was forgotten and it was thought that they earned their name because they ate hashish.

Hashbury. Haight-Ashbury District in San Francisco.

Hashish. Originally a general Arabic term for grass or fodder, medicinal herbs, or weeds. Hashish evolved as a nickname for "the herb"—cannabis. It now refers to resin-covered flowers or bracts of cannabis, which generally contain more THC than other parts of the plant.

Hashish Club. *See* Club des Haschischins.

Hassle. Inconvenience; problem; unpleasant situation; difficulty in buying marihuana.
1966: "It reaches the point where it's not worth the hassle." (*Village Voice*, December 1, p. 21).
1974: ". . . the hassles it took to get that weed to your living room." (*High Times*, vol. 1, no. 1, p. 8).

Hay. Marihuana. *See also* Hot Hay.
1934: "The leaves and blossoms are then packed in pocket-sized

tobacco tins which retail at \$3 to \$5 each and contain enough 'hay' to make thirty or forty cigarettes, one of which is enough to intoxicate the smoker." (*New York Times*, September 16, p. 21).

1942: "Hay." (Berrey and Bark, *Thesaurus*, p. 474).

1949: "Hay." (Monteleone, *Criminal Slang*, p. 114).

1961: "Hay." (Partridge, *Dictionary*, p. 324).

Hay Burner. Marihuana user.

1943: "The 'snowbird' (cocaine sniffer) and 'hay-burner' (marihuana smoker) are carried off into a state equivalent to deep alcoholic intoxication." (*Life*, July 19, p. 85).

1949: "Hay burner." (Monteleone, *Criminal Slang*, p. 114).

Hay Butt. Marihuana cigarette.

1942: "Hay butt." (Berrey and Bark, *Thesaurus*, p. 476).

1949: "Hay butt." (Monteleone, *Criminal Slang*, p. 114).

Hay Head. Marihuana user.

1949: "Hay head." (Monteleone, *Criminal Slang*, p. 114).

1955: "Hay head." (Braddy, "Narcotic Argot," p. 87).

Head. Chronic marihuana user or chronic user of any drug. Someone so involved with marihuana it has become an important part of his life.

1937: "These were the real heads." (Ric, *Esquire*, p. 192).

1956: "Being a 'head' is being part of a whole new culture." (Longstreet, *Real Jazz*, p. 147).

1959: "When the marijuana head (vipers, we called them in the thirties) or the hype turns on . . . " (Lipton, *Holy Barbarians*, p. 171).

Head Drug. Drug affecting the mind, primarily through altering consciousness.

Head Gear. Drug paraphernalia, for example, pipes, papers, clips.

Head Shop. Store selling paraphernalia for smoking marihuana or other drug use.

1967: "Head shop." (Brown, *Hippies*, p. 218).

1968: "A head shop is where one buys the accessories of the psychedelic experience." (*New York Times*, January 11, p. 18/1).

1974: ". . . a friend who runs a headshop . . ." (*High Times*, vol. 1, no. 2, p. 7).

Heat. Police.

1969: "They never threatened to call the heat." (*Time*, September 26, p. 73).

Heat's On. Police are looking for drug user to arrest.

Heavy. Profound; considerable; potent.

Heavy Hash. Potent hashish.

Heeled. Having money.

Hemp. 1. General name for many different bast fibers, for example, jute, sisal. Hemp proper refers to bast fiber of *Cannabis sativa*, the marihuana plant. (*See* below for derivation of word.) 2. Marihuana. 3. Cowboy term for rope. Derived from best ropes being made of hemp fiber.

Due to the unsurpassed strength of its fiber, hemp was a highly valued material in the manufacture of many items, especially rope. Because most ropes were made from hemp, it came to be synonymous with rope, particularly the rope used to hang those found guilty of various crimes.

The English word *hemp* is derived from the Indo-European Sanskrit, *sana*, meaning a hollow, reedlike plant or cane; Greek *kannabos* and *kannabis* refers to a bow string (*bios*) made from hemp (cane).

The root *an* recurs in all Indo-European and modern Semitic languages but has undergone various changes. For example, the Greek *k* became *c* in Latin (*cannabis*), *ch* in modern French (*chanvre*), and *h* or *k* in various European languages, for example, *hanaf* (old high German), *hanef* (middle high German), and *hanf* (modern German); and the *a* occasionally became *e*, while the *f* became *p*, for example, *hennep*, *kennep* (Dutch), *haenep* (old English). The change from *n* to *m* resulted in *hamp* in Danish and *hemp* in Anglo-Saxon.

Hemp fiber ceased to be a valuable economic commodity in the post-Civil war era after the introduction of wire baling. Current use of the word is generally in reference to marihuana.

1931: ". . . restrictions respecting the smoking of 'hemp' . . ." (Stanley, "Marihuana," p. 254).

1952: ". . . three sticks of hemp." (Mandell, *Flee the Angry Strangers*, p. 229).

1967: "They live a big hemp-crazy myth." (Chaplin, *Grass*, p. 157).

1976: "I am out in my hemp every day." (*High Times*, November, p. 102).

Hemp, Barren. Male cannabis plant.

Hemp, Carl (Charle, Churle, Karl). Female hemp plant. Because the female cannabis plant lived longer and produced the coarser fiber of the two sexes of the cannabis plant, it was mistakenly thought to be the male (Carl). The terms *Carl*, *Charle*, and such were used as synonyms for stubbornness.

1722: "You have a stalk of carle hemp in you." (Quoted by *Oxford English Dictionary*, 1973, p. 1289).

Hemp Committee. Vigilantes bent on hanging (hemping) someone.

Hempen Collar. Hangman's noose.

Hempen Cravat. Hangman's noose.

Hempen Fever. Death. To die of hempen fever was to be hanged. The victim was sometimes said to have been given a chance to look at the sky.

1839: "Husbands died of hempen fever." (Ainsworth, *Jack Sheppard*, quoted by Farmer and Henley, *Slang*, vol. 2, p. 302).

Hempen Fortune. Bad luck; reference to being hanged.

Hempen Garter. Hangman's noose.

Hempen Halter. Hangman's noose.

Hempen Necklace. Hangman's noose.

1886: "Nothing but the immediate prospect of a hempen necklace would extort that." (Braddon, *Mohawks*, quoted by Farmer and Henley, *Slang*, vol. 2, p. 302).

Hempen Necktie. Hangman's noose.

1940: "We wanted to lynch Frank Canton, and if we had been allowed to hand him a hemp necktie right then, it would have saved a heap of good men.") Barber and Walker, *Longest Rope*, p. 34, quoted by Mathews, *Dictionary*, p. 940).

Hemp (en) Party. A lynching.

1892: "If the incendiarist is found, a hemp party may yet result." (*Columbus Ohio Dispatch*, Dec. 6, p. 1/2.).

Hempen Seed. Disreputable person.

Hempen Widow. Wife of a man who has been hanged.

Hep, Hip. Aware; knowledgeable; sophisticated.

Herb. Marihuana.

1970: "Herb." (*Current Slang*, vol. 5, no. 2, p. 8).

1972: "Herb." (Claerbaut, *Black Jargon*, p. 68).

1976: "Bob smokes about a pound of marihuana or 'herb' a week."
(*High Times*, September, p. 47).
1980: "I have to smoke Hawaiian or Thai herb to do this." (Novak,
High Culture, p. 255).

Herodotus. "Father of History." Greek historian. First (A.D. 450) to
describe the use of marihuana for psychoactive properties. Herodotus
relates how the Scythians, a group of nomadic Arian warriors, threw
marihuana seeds (probably bracts) on hot coals and inhaled the fumes
as part of funeral purification rites:

> "The Scythians then take the seeds of this hemp and, creeping under the
> mats, they throw them on the red-hot stones; and being so thrown, they
> smoulder and send forth so much steam that no Greek vapor bath could
> surpass it. The Scythians howl in their joy at their vapor bath." (*Histories*,
> 5:72).

High. Euphoric; intoxicated; drugged; exhilarated. The most frequent
term used to describe the pleasurable effects of marihuana. Previously
used as synonym for alcohol intoxication.
1936: "When I Get Low, I Get High." Song recorded by Chick Webb.
1937: "When they get high on the stuff you can write your own
ticket." (Anon., "Marihuana," p. 184).
1938: "This 'high' effect is present when some object that is being
observed grows smaller and smaller until only a blurred spot
remains." (Yawger, "Marihuana," p. 355).
1938: "A smoker is high when contentment creeps over him."
(Berger, *New Yorker*, March 12, p. 47).
1944: "I lit up for this big deal and was higher than those mountains
before we even got there. . . . By the time the bus creaked into
town I was so high on the weed I couldn't tell which Trinidad
we were in." (Mezzrow and Wolfe, *Really the Blues*, p. 135).
1952: "Only the men got high." (Mandell, *Flee the Angry Strangers*,
p. 240).
1953: "Would you like to get high?" (Burroughs, *Junkie*, p. 33).
1955: "I was kind of high but they didn't notice." (Ellson, *Rock*,
p. 29).
1956: "High—a state in which time seems to stand still, where the top
of the head is filled with all of heaven, and everything seems
easy to do, better, stronger, and longer." (Longstreet, *Real Jazz*,
p. 144).
1958: "I'm as high as a Georgia pine." (Hughes and Bontemps, *Negro
Folklore*, p. 484).

1969: "Gangster was sure a whore's high." (Iceberg Slim, *Pimp*, p. 152).

1974: "Most people smoke to achieve a certain level of high which they know to be just right for them." (Isyurhash and Rusoff, *Gourmet*, p. 17).

Hippies. Individuals following a counterculture way of life based on renunciation of material things and believing it possible to achieve deep insight into life through use of drugs like marihuana. Hippies flourished during the 1960s.

Hit. 1. Purchase marihuana. 2. Smoke marihuana. 3. Take a deep inhalation from a marihuana cigarette. Originally an intense reaction from narcotics or purchase of narcotics (1940s). *See also* Blast, Toke.

1952: "Take harder hits on it; don't sip it like you're scared." (Mandell, *Flee the Angry Strangers*, p. 241).

1962: "He gagged down on the smoke to hold it in. . . . 'Take a good hit, Tari.' " (Pritchie, *Savage Kick*, p. 89).

1967: "I take a deep hit of the acrid smoke." (Simmons, *Marihuana*, p. 22).

1971: "He took a big hit through the mouth of the chillum." (Coyote Man, *Buzz*, p. 5).

1978: "Two hits of Colombian is enough for me." (*High Times*, July, p. 41).

1979: "Oaxacan was one of my early hits." (Goldman, *Grass Roots*, p. 40).

Hit the hay. Smoke marihuana. Possibly a pun on the same expression meaning to go to sleep.

Hit the moon. Very high* as a result of smoking marihuana.

HOG. Hash, O, Grass. Term for marihuana used by American soldier in Vietnam.

1968: "HOG." (*Rolling Stone*, November 9, p. 5).

Hoka toka. Smoking marihuana; having a toke.*

Holding. Possessing marihuana or other drugs for sale.

1938: "Hold." (Maurer, "Argot of Underworld," p. 185).

1952: "Are you holding?" (Lannoy and Masterson, "Hophead Jargon," p. 24).

1953: "Are you holding?" (Burroughs, *Junkie*, p. 15).

1956: "Are you holding?" (Hunter, *Second Ending*, p. 244).

1962: "What are you holding?" (Pritchie, *Savage Kick*, p. 120).

1968: "I don't know nobody that's holding." (Bloomquist, *Mari-huana*, p. 54).

1968: "If they catch you holding." (*Marihuana Review*, vol. 1, no. 1, p. 3).

Home-grown. Domestic marihuana. Marihuana grown in someone's home or backyard.

1976: "The Association is offering $40 a pound for homegrown." (*High Times*, November, p. 96).

Honey Oil. Hash oil.

1976: "There seem to be many different types of hash oils being marketed today—cherry Leb, Afghani, honey oil, Indian oil, etc." (*High Times*, July, p. 16).

Hooch. Marihuana. Originally alcohol.

Hookah. Water pipe for smoking marihuana, hashish, tobacco, and so on. Smoke is first drawn through water and cooled, making it less harsh.

Hop Party. Marihuana party. Originally an opium-smoking party.

1938: "Hop party." (Walton, *Marihuana*, p. 195).

Hophead. Marihuana or drug user. Originally an opium user.

1953: "All these hopheads really go for it." (Manning, *Reefer*, p. 47).

Horrors. Paranoia concerning arrest for marihuana possession.

1952: "I've got the horrors something awful." (Mandell, *Flee the Angry Strangers*, p. 132).

1962: "Don't get the horrors." (Pritchie, *Savage Kick*, p. 23).

Hot Box. Room filled with marihuana smoke.

Hot Hay. Marihuana.

1951: "Other slang names include 'weed,' 'hay,' or 'hot hay.' " (*San Diego Evening Tribune*, July 15, p. A17/1).

Hot Sticks. Marihuana cigarettes. *See also* Stick.

Hotel Lauzun (Hotel Pimodan). Scene of the monthly meetings of the Club des Haschischins.* Located in Paris's Latin Quarter.

Hotel Pimodan. *See* Hotel Lauzun.

House Hearings on Marihuana. U.S. Congress, House of Representatives, Hearings on the Taxation of Marihuana, H.R. 6385, House Committee on Ways and Means, 75th Congress, 1937. Chairman, Robert Doughton.

Hearings to determine whether marihuana should be outlawed. These hearings resulted in the passage of the Marihuana Tax Act in 1937.

Hubble Bubble. Water-cooled pipe. *See* Hookah.

Hung up. 1. Dependent on drugs. 2. Bothered by problems.

Hunk. A quarter-ounce or more of hashish.
1971: "Hunk." (Eschholz and Rosa, "Slang," p. 14).

Hurds. Refuse left after hemp* fiber is removed from its stalk. During the turn of the century, the U.S. Department of Agriculture proposed using hemp hurds as a substitute for paper.

Hustle. To sell drugs.
1967: "I started to hustle pot." (Thomas, *Mean Streets*, p. 215).

Hypnotics. Drugs causing sleep and confusion.

I

Ice Bag, Ice Pack. Potent marihuana allegedly smuggled into California inside boxes of frozen lettuce.
1969: "Ice Pack was selling for $300." (Margolis and Clorfene, *Grass*, p. 121).

In. Intoxicated with marihuana.
1938: ". . . being 'in,' meaning the subject is under the influence." (Yawger, "Marihuana," p. 355).

Incense. Marihuana.
1969: "Torch a coupla sticks of incense." (Iceberg Slim, *Pimp*, p. 152).

Indian Bay. Marihuana.

Indian Hay. Marihuana.
1936: "The drug and cigarettes containing it are known as . . . 'Indian hay' . . ." (Spencer, "Marihuana," p. 300).
1938: "The drug is known by many different names, such as 'Indian hay' . . ." (Yawger, "Marihuana," p. 351).
1943: "Marihuana may be called 'Indian hay.' " (*Time*, July 19, p. 54).
1949: "Indian hay." (Monteleone, *Criminal Slang*, p. 129).

Indian Hemp. Marihuana.

1937: "A number of other names are also used, such as 'Indian hemp'
    . . ." (Weber, "Mary Warner," p. 77).

Indian Hemp Drugs Commission. First (1893-1894) government-spon-
sored study of the physical, mental, and moral effects of marihuana
(called *bhang, ganja,* and *charas*). The commission consisted of seven
examiners (four British, three Indian) appointed by the British viceroy
to India. The data consisted of written or oral answers submitted by
1,193 "witnesses" to seven questions. In general, the commission concluded that "moderate" use of marihuana was not harmful, but failed
to define what it meant by "moderate." For its time, a landmark
study, impartial and objective, but unacceptable by present-day scientific standards. The report filled seven volumes and was 3,281 pages
long.

Indian Oil. Hash oil.

Indian Rope. Potent hashish from India.

Indian Weed. Marihuana.
1937: "It has been called Indian weed because its strong pungent odor
    resembles that of burning hay." (Weber, "Mary Warner," p. 78).

Into. 1. Using drugs. 2. Concerned or involved with something.

Isomerize. To rearrange atoms in a molecule so that physical and
chemical properties are changed, although molecular weight remains
the same, for example, CBD can be isomerized to THC.

Isomerizer. Device for changing other cannabinoids into THC, thereby
increasing the potency of marihuana.

J

J (Jay). Marihuana cigarette.
1968: "In Vietnam you buy ten already rolled Js for 100 piastres
    (88¢)." (*Rolling Stone,* November 9, p. 5).
1970: ". . . smoke a marihuana joint, 'j's' as the joints were nick-
    named . . ." (Kaplan, "Marijuana," p. 26).
1970: "Jay." (Gardner, "Slang," p. 20).
1971: "Smoke the J until it goes out." (Coyote Man, *Buzz,* p. 86).

J (Jay) Pipe. Pipe for smoking marihuana.

J (Jay) Smoke. Marihuana.

Jacked up. Under the influence of drugs, including marihuana.
1935: "Jacked up." (Pollock, *Underworld Speaks*, p. 12).

Jag. 1. Under the influence of marihuana. 2. Uncontrollable behavior,
for example, "laughing jag"—uncontrollable laughter.
1928: "One cigaret will produce a tremendous jag, almost a spree."
        (*Chicago Tribune*, July 1, p. 12).
1943: "Two or three long puffs usually suffice after a while to produce
        a light jag." (*Time*, July 19, p. 54).
1944: "One man suddenly got a 'laughing jag.' " (*La Guardia Report*,
        p. 43).

Jahooby. Marihuana.
1956: "You can't get hooked on jahooby." (Duke, *Sideman*, p. 277).

Jamaican. Potent marihuana from Jamaica.
1974: "Most people now place Colombian at the top, with Jamaican
        and Mexican placing two and three, respectively." (*High Times*,
        vol. 1, no. 1, p. 9).

Jane's Better Half. Marihuana user.
1959: "Jane's better half." (Schmidt, *Narcotics*, p. 93).

Jefferson Airplane. Device for holding the burning butt of a marihuana
cigarette. *See also* Bridge, Clip.
1967: "The butt, or roach, is tucked into the Y of a split paper match
        Mizou students call a Jefferson airplane." (*Look*, August 18,
        p. 16).
1969: "Split the match down the middle almost to the head, put the
        roach in between and hold the ends closed. This is called an air-
        plane, or Jefferson Airplane." (Margolis and Clorfene, *Grass*,
        p. 109).

Jersey Green. Domestic marihuana grown in New Jersey.

Jingo. Marihuana.
1968: "Jingo." (Dawtry, *Drug Abuse*, p. 91).

Jive. 1. Marihuana. 2. Insincerity.
1936: "All the Jive Is Gone." Song recorded by Pha Terrell.
1952: "It's only guage he's on, a little jive." (Mandell, *Flee the Angry
        Strangers*, p. 24).
1960: "Let's turn on a little jive here." (De Mexico, *Marijuana Girl*,
        p. 120).

1962: "It's coming on thick in my throat, Howie. It's good jive."
(Pritchie, *Savage Kick*, p. 27).
1969: "Jive." (Williams, *Narcotics*, p. 138).

Jive Sticks. Marihuana cigarettes.
1969: "Jive stick." (Williams, *Narcotics*, p. 113).
1977: "Jive stick." (Lentini, *Vice*, p. 138).

Johnson. Marihuana.
1970: "Johnson." (*Current Slang*, vol. 5, no. 2, p. 9).

Joint. 1. Hand-rolled marihuana cigarette. 2. Paraphernalia for narcotics
injection. 3. A place to live. 4. Jail. 5. A penis.
1954: "When the amount has been broken up into cigarettes (. . .
'sticks' or 'joints') . . ." (Bevan, *Everybody's*, June 12, p. 11).
1956: "Two or three people can get high on one joint." (Longstreet,
Real Jazz, p. 146).
1956: "The first time I gave you a joint, it was right on the street."
(Hunter, *Second Ending*, p. 94).
1959: "Joint: A place, a penis, a marijuana cigarette, preferably a
combination of the three." (Lipton, *Holy Barbarians*, p. 355).
1966: "The profit remains as tempting at every stage of dealing—
probably around six exchanged from field to joint." (*Village
Voice*, December 1, p. 20).
1966: "They shared the joint while walking, speaking not another
word." (Farina, *Been Down So Long*, p. 112).
1967: "A joint today, they think means a junkie tomorrow." (*Time*,
September 26, p. 70).
1969: "She started rolling a joint." (Iceberg Slim, *Pimp*, p. 152).
1977: "He was standing there smoking a joint." (Rettig et al., *Manny*,
p. 32).
1979: "Tony smiles and offers them a joint." (Goldman, *Grass Roots*,
p. 24).

Jolt. Initial effect of marihuana or other psychoactive drug.

Joy Smoke. Marihuana.
1943: "Cigarettes made from it are called 'joy smokes.' " (*Time*,
July 19, p. 54).

Joy Stick. 1. Marihuana cigarette. 2. Opium pipe.

Juane. Marihuana; abbreviation of Mary Jane or marijuana.
1934: "I had a glass of beer on top of the piano and a half-smoked
juane on the side." (Wylie, *Finnley Wren*, p. 51).

Juanita. Marihuana.

1917: "They have had no importations under the name of Indian Hemp, *Cannabis indica*, Marihuana, or Juanita." (Smith, Dept. of Agriculture, p. 8).

1955: ". . . Mexican plant known as 'D. Juanita'. . ." (de Farias, "Maconha," p. 5).

Juanita Weed. Marihuana.

Ju Ju. Marihuana.

1940: "I knew a guy who smoked ju jus. Three highballs, and three sticks of tea and it took a pipe wrench to get him off the chandelier." (Chandler, *Farewell, My Lovely*, p. 60).

Junkerman. Marihuana smoker.

1945: "In New Orleans smokers of the drug are called "junkermen.' " (Saxon, *Gumbo*, p. 461).

K

Kaif, Keef, Kheef, Kif. Marihuana; hashish.

Kanjac. Marihuana.

1925: ". . . the plant known as Cannabis Indica or Cannabis America or Indian Hemp (Haschisch), or in the vernacular expression: Marijuana, Ganja or Kanjac." (*Panama Canal Zone Report*, p. 1).

Kee, Key, Ki. Kilogram (2.2 pounds) of marihuana or hashish.

1968: "It is still possible to grab a New York flight with two 'keys' of grass (about $300)." (*Rolling Stone*, October 18, p. 5).

Keep off the grass. Don't use marihuana.

Keyed up. High on marihuana.

1972: "Keyed up." (Folb, *Black Argot*, p. 88).

Kick. 1. Excitement; reaction; sensation; elation from drug use. 2. To give up drug use.

1938: "A high-school girl had heard some whisperings concerning the 'kick' offered by the new kind of cigarette." (Yawger, "Marihuana," p. 356).

1955: ". . . the best kicks I have known." (Braddy, "Anonymous Verses," p. 132).

Kick Stick. Marihuana cigarette.

1967: "Joints are pulled out of the brims of hats and soon there is no noise except the music and the steady hiss of cats blasting away on kick sticks." (Thomas, *Mean Streets*, p. 155).

Killer, Killer Stick. Marihuana cigarette.

1943: "Cigarettes made from it are called killers." (*Time*, July 19, p. 54).

1967: "But so many myths about marihuana as the 'killer weed' have been spread." (*Newsweek*, July 24, p. 46).

Kiss Mary Jane. Smoke marihuana.

1959: "Kiss Mary Jane." (Schmidt, *Narcotics*, p. 97).

Kite. Ounce of marihuana.

Knock yourself crazy. Smoke marihuana.

1938: "Knock ourselves crazy." (Walton, *Marihuana*, p. 195).

1941: "Knocking Myself Out." Song recorded by Lil Green.

Kona Gold. Potent marihuana from the Hawaiian island of Kona.

1976: "This Kona Gold plant sure glistens with resin under our hot Hawaiian sun." (*High Times*, September, p. 12).

1980: "On Kona Gold you really can't even think because you're so gone." (Novak, *High Culture*, p. 191).

Kona Kona. *See* Kona Gold.

L

La Guardia Report (The Marihuana Problem in the City of New York). First detailed sociological and clinical study of the effects of marihuana. The report was initiated by the New York Academy of Medicine in 1938 at the request of New York Mayor Fiorello La Guardia. The study was conducted between 1940 and 1941. Field studies were conducted by undercover New York police officers in Harlem. The report was published in 1944.

Lamarck, Jean. French biologist who contended that there was more than one species of cannabis. Lamarck reserved the term *Cannabis sativa* for cannabis grown in Europe and gave the term *Cannabis* *indica* to the variety that grew in India and contained more of the psychotomimetic material.

Lame. 1. Someone who doesn't smoke marihuana. 2. Weak; feeble.

Lard. Police officer.

Laughing Grass. Marihuana.

Laughing Jag. *See* Jag.

Laughing Tobacco. Marihuana.

Lay. To sell marihuana or offer it as an unsolicited gift.
1960: "We got plenty of pot and I'll lay some on you." (De Mexico, *Marijuana Girl*, p. 100).
1961: "He'd lay a few joints on the cats and they'd lay a little bread on him." (Hughes, *Fantastic Lodge*, p. 145).
1968: ". . . some marijuana that has just been laid on her by a friend." (Gross, *Flower People*, p. 21).
1972: "Petie brings out some grass and mentions, in passing, that 'someone laid it on me the other day.' " (Cavan, *Hippies*, p. 132).
1974: "He will roll up, share a joint with you, lay some on at a decent price . . ." (Isyurhash and Rusoff, *Gourmet*, p. 36).

Laying down the hustle. Selling marihuana. *See also* Hustle.
1943: "Are you laying down the hustle?" (*Time*, July 19, p. 54).

Leary, Dr. Timothy. Harvard psychologist. Leary was a pioneer in LSD and other drug-related research. He was fired from Harvard because of his drug studies. He was once known as the "high priest of pot."

Leaves. Marihuana.

Leb, Lebanese. Hashish from Lebanon.
1975: "Lebanese will remain a connoisseur item." (*High Times*, October, p. 43).

Le Dain Commission. Named after Gerald Le Dain, chairman of the Canadian Commission of Inquiry into the Nonmedical Use of Drugs. The commission concluded that marihuana was a relatively benign drug.

LEMAR. First (1965) organized effort to work for legalization of marihuana. Founded by a lawyer, the movement challenged the constitutionality of marihuana laws. Members included eminent "beatniks" such as Allen Ginsburg. The first university chapter was based in Buffalo, New York. The movement disbanded without having any impact on marihuana legislation.

Lemonade. Weak marihuana.
1980: "Really bad grass we called 'lemonade.' " (Novak, *High Culture*, p. 168).

Leno. Marihuana cigarette (Chicano), literally "piece of firewood."
1955: "Leno." (Braddy, "Narcotic Argot," p. 87).

Leper Grass. Potent marihuana from Colombia.

Let it all hang out. Hide nothing; be honest.

Licata, Victor. Convicted murderer. Licata was said to have axed his mother, father, brothers, and sister to death while under the influence of marihuana. The family had history of insanity, and Licata had been committed to an institution a year earlier, but his parents had had him released, claiming they could take better care of him. Licata was found not guilty by reason of insanity. In 1950 he hanged himself.

Lid. Small, clear plastic bag containing about one to two ounces of loose, uncleaned marihuana. The bag is wrapped in thick roll and sealed with masking or Scotch tape. It will make about forty marihuana cigarettes.
1967: "In the Hashbury, grass can be had for $10 to $15 a 'lid.' " (*Time*, July 7, p. 21).
1968: "Keys are going for around $180. Lids are $10." (*Grass Profit Review*, June 10, no. 6, p. 1).
1972: "He bought a lid of grass for $20 but it was 75 percent straw." (Hall, *Heads*, pp. 65-66).
1979: "I gotta get fifty a lid to make any money." (Goldman, *Grass Roots*, p. 24).

Lid Action. Purchase of a lid* of marihuana.

Lie in state with the girls. Smoke marihuana. From the names, Mary Jane, Mary Warner, and such given to marihuana.
1959: "Lie in state with the girls." (Schmidt, *Narcotics*, p. 101).

Lightning Hashish. Potent hashish used by dealers for their own personal enjoyment.

Linnaeus, Carolus. Swedish botanist who gave the marihuana plant its present botanical name, *Cannabis sativa* ("cultivated cane").

Lipton's. Weak marihuana (1940s). Term was probably derived from the tea brand. Marihuana is also known as tea.*

Liquid Grass. THC.*
1971: "Liquid grass." (Eschholz and Rosa, "Slang," p. 15).

Lit Up. Under the influence of marihuana or narcotics.

Loaded. Intoxicated.
1976: "I was getting loaded on weed regularly." (Sutter, "Righteous Dope Fiend," p. 192).

Loco Weed. Marihuana. Not to be confused with plant (*Astrafulus mollisimus*) also known as loco weed that makes cattle sick.
1931: "It is sometimes mentioned in the law as 'loco weed' because of its inebriant effect upon men and cattle." (Stanley, "Marihuana," p. 254).
1936: "The drug and cigarettes containing it are known as . . . 'loco weed.' " (Spencer, "Marihuana," p. 300).
1937: "A number of other names are also used such as . . . loco weed." (Weber, "Mary Warner," p. 77).
1937: "The worst thing about that loco weed is the way kids go for them." (Anon., "Marihuana," p. 184).
1969: "It is commonly known as hemp, Indian hemp, loco weed, or marihuana." (Williams, *Narcotics*, p. 140).

Log. Marihuana cigarette.

Long. Tightly packed marihuana.
1968: "Cans are of two sizes, short (loosely packed) and long (tightly packed)." (Bloomquist, *Marihuana*, p. 54).

Loose. Relaxed.

Love Weed. Marihuana. From marihuana's alleged aphrodisiac properties.
1943: "Marihuana may be called . . . love weed." (*Time*, July 19, p. 54).

Lover. Marihuana smoker.
1959: "Lover." (Schmidt, *Narcotics*, p. 103).

Lozerose. *See* Lozies.

Lozies. Marihuana.
1946: "The words lozies and lozeerose were coined so guys could refer to my gauge without having anybody else dig it." (Mezzrow and Wolfe, *Really the Blues*, p. 211).

Ludlow, Fitz Hugh (1836-1870). First American author to write a full-length book about marihuana (*The Hasheesh Eater: Being Passages from* *the Life of a Pythagorean*, 1857). He is also the author of the first book on marihuana in English. The book deals with his experiences with large doses of cannabis extract (Tilden's extract) obtained from an apothecary shop in Poughkeepsie, New York. Ludlow's book is now considered a minor classic of its type.

> There are two facts which I have verified as universal by repeated experiment, which fall into their place here as aptly as they can in the course of my narrative: 1st. At two different times, when body and mind are apparently in precisely analogous states, when all circumstances, exterior and interior, do not differ tangibly in the smallest respect, the same dose of the same preparation of hasheesh will frequently produce diametrically opposite effects. Still further, I have taken at one time a pill of thirty grains, which hardly gave a perceptible phenomenon, and at another, when my dose had been but half that quantity, I have suffered the agonies of a martyr, or rejoiced in a perfect phrensy.
>
> So exceedingly variable are its results, that, long before I abandoned the indulgence, I took each successive bolus with the consciousness that I was daring an uncertainty as tremendous as the equipoise between hell and heaven. Yet the fascination employed Hope as its advocate, and won the suit. 2nd. If, during the ecstasy of hasheesh delirium, another dose, however small—yes, though it be no larger than half a pea—be employed to prolong the condition, such agony will inevitably ensue as will make the soul shudder at its own possibility of endurance without annihilation. By repeated experiments, which now occupy the most horrible place upon my catalogue of horrible remembrances, have I proved that, among all the variable phenomena of hasheesh, this alone stands unvarying. (Ludlow, *Hasheesh Eater*, p. 66).

Lumber. Stems of the marihuana plant.

Lusher. Alcoholic who mixes marihuana with alcohol.
1955: "Lusher." (Braddy, "Narcotic Argot," p. 87).

M

M. 1. Marihuana. 2. Morphine.
1956: "You don't need a shooting gallery for a stick of M." (Hunter, *Second Ending*, p. 94).

M'M's. Marihuana munchies. *See* Munchies.
1971: "M.M.s." (Eschholz and Rosa, "Slang," p. 16).

Mach. Marihuana.

Machu Picchu. Potent marihuana from Peru.

Maggie, Megg. Marihuana.
1959: "Maggie." (Schmidt, *Narcotics*, p. 109).

Make a buy. Purchase marihuana.
1967: "A pot smoker turned loose in a city where he knows no one,
seeking a can of stuff, will be able to make a buy before night-
fall." (Rosevear, *Pot*, p. 27).

Man, The. 1. Seller of marihuana. Possibly originating from "The Old
Man of the Mountain"; 2. Police officer.
1932: "The Man from Harlem." Title of song recorded by Cab
Calloway.
1955: "I bet they're capping right now from their man." (Braddy,
"Anonymous Verses," p. 133).
1956: "The Man is always on the scene ready to oblige." (Hunter,
Second Ending, p. 250).

Man from Montana. Marihuana seller.
1955: ". . . the 'man from Montana' (a variant of 'The Old Man of the
mountain') . . ." (Braddy, "Anonymous Verses," p. 133).

Manicure. To remove stems and seeds from crude marihuana.

Manicured. Cleaned marihuana.
1968: "A portion is removed from the stash, manicured, and rolled
into joints." (Bloomquist, *Marihuana*, p. 58).

Manhattan Silver, Manhattan White. Light-colored marihuana allegedly
grown in sewers of New York as a result of being flushed down the
toilet to avoid possession arrest. Considered to be very potent. Silver
color is due to growth in absence of sun preventing photosynthesis.
A hoax.
1976: "Enterprising dealers often use the epithet 'Manhattan Silver'
to boost sales of any light-colored grass they may have in
stock." (*High Times*, March, p. 12).

Marfil. Brand of marihuana cigarette paper.

Mari, Mary. Marihuana.
1933: ". . . locally designated by such names as . . . Mari." (Hayes and
Bowery, "Marihuana," p. 1087).
1949: "Mari." (Monteleone, *Criminal Slang*, p. 153).

Mariahuana. Marihuana.
1931: "Mariahuana." (Fossier, "Marihuana Menace," p. 247).

Marihuana. Mixture of leaves, flowers, and stems from the plant *Cannabis sativa* or *Cannabis indica*. It has the potential for intoxication due to its THC content.

Up until the 1970s, marihuana available in the United States contained about 1 percent THC. THC content has subsequently increased so that in many cases it is as high as 4 percent. The average marihuana cigarette contains about 500 mg. of marihuana and about 5 to 20 mg. THC.

When smoked, only about 50 percent THC reaches the lungs; 25 percent of THC is lost in conbustion, 5 percent is lost in uninhaled smoke, and 20 percent is trapped in the butt (roach*).

Effects of marihuana are observed at doses as low as 25 mcg. (one mcg. is 1/1000 of one mg.) per kg (1,000 g. or 2.2 lbs.) of body weight. Intense hallucinations occur around 250 mcg. per kg. No deaths due to an overdose of marihuana have ever been reported.

The etymology of the word is unknown. It is most likely derived from the Mexican-Spanish *mariguana*, meaning "intoxicant." However, mention of the term *marihuana* in the title of a medical thesis written in 1886 (see below) predates reference to *mariguana* (see below).

Another frequently mentioned origin is that the word was formed from the Mexican names "Maria" *y* (and) "Juan" or "Juanita" (Mary and Jane). However, this doesn't account for how or why it came to be called by these names in the first place.

1886: *La Marihuana. Breve Estudio de esta Planta. (Marihuana, Brief Study of the Plant.* Thesis written by Perez Genaro).

1894: "(The) 'toloachi' (and) the 'mariguan' are used by discarded women for the purpose of wreaking a terrible revenge upon recreant lovers." (*Scribner's Magazine*, May, p. 596/2).

1897: "The natives of Mexico are fond of a weed called mariguana, for mixing with their tobacco in their cigarettes, which when it is smoked and inhaled by them is said to produce a hilarious spirit in the smoker." (*St. Louis Globe-Democrat*, November 18, p. 1).

1917: "In the border States, and especially Texas, in the vicinity of San Antonio, there is considerable marihuana grown." (Smith, Dept. of Agriculture, p. 4).

1923: "Marijuana is a form of drug that brings fake heart to the user." (Smith, *Little Tigress*, p. 102-3).

1925: "In reference to investigations directed through Committee as

to the use of 'Mariahuana,' it appears that there is very little
information on the subject." (*Panama Canal Zone Report*, p. 3).
1928: "You can grow enough marihuana in a window-box to drive the
whole population of the United States staring raving mad."
(Black, *Dope*, p. 42).

Marihuana and Health Reporting Act (PL 91-296, 1970). Law requiring secretary of Health, Education, and Welfare to report annually
concerning current information on the health consequences of marihuana.

Marihuana Tax Act (PL 75-238, 1937). U.S. federal antimarihuana
law requiring anyone buying marihuana to obtain a tax stamp.

Mary. *See* Mari.

Mary and Johnny. Marihuana.
1935: "Mary and Johnny." (Pollock, *Underworld Speaks*, p. 15).

Mary Ann. Marihuana.

Mary Anner. Marihuana.

Mary Jane, Mary Juana, M.J. Marihuana.
1928: ". . . mariajuana—Mary Jane—the Mexican drug." (*Chicago
Tribune*, July 1, p. 12).
1934: "In short, a 'muggles,' 'weed,' or 'mootie,' cannabis indica,
Indian hemp, or, to give it its Mexican name, marijuana, which
translated into English just means Mary Jane!" (De Lenoir,
Hundredth Man, p. 220).
1937: "Command a person 'high' on 'mu' or 'muggles' or 'Mary Jane'
to crawl on the floor and bark like a dog, and he will do it without a thought of the idiocy of the action." (Anslinger, "Marihuana," p. 152).
1937: "They are spoken of as . . . 'Mary Janes.' " (Anon., "Marihuana," p. 184).
1959: "Blues for Mary Jane." Song recorded by Stan Getz.
1969: "Mary Jane." (Williams, *Narcotics*, p. 114).
1971: "Most of the new people who move Maryjane aren't getting
rich from their deals." (Coyote Man, *Buzz*, p. 90).

Mary Warner. Marihuana. *See also* Mary Weaver, Mary Werner.
1933: "Mary Warner . . . this name is probably arrived at because the
purchaser is unable to pronounce correctly the Mexican name
'marihuana.' " (Hayes and Bowery, "Marihuana," p. 1087).

1938: "The drug is known by many different names such as . . . 'Mary Warner.' " (Yawger, "Marihuana," p. 351).

Mary Weaver. Marihuana.
1937: "Some people call it . . . 'Mary Weaver.' " (Anslinger, "Marihuana," p. 150).

Mary Werner. Marihuana.
1949: "Mary Werner." (Monteleone, *Criminal Slang*, p. 153).

Matchbox. About one-fifth of a lid.* It makes up to five to ten cigarettes.
1967: "A matchbox of the stuff goes for $5." (Brown, *Hippies*, p. 189).
1967: ". . . $5 for a matchboxful that can produce about 10 joints." (*Time*, July 7, p. 21).

Maui (Wowie). Marihuana from Hawaiian island of Maui. Potent.
1978: "Better grass is grown in Hawaii (Maui Wowie, Kona Gold, etc.)." (*Playboy*, September, p. 220).

Meet. Meeting place between drug buyer and seller.
1955: "I went on to the meet." (Braddy, "Anonymous Verses," p. 13).

Megg. *See* Maggie.

Mellow. Pleasant, nice, enjoyable, calm, relaxed.
1935: "The Stuff Is Here and Its Mellow." Song recorded by Cleo Brown.
1938: "Jack, I'm Mellow." Song recorded by Trixie Smith.
1971: "Everybody was too mellow to notice that she bogarted the J." (Coyote Man, *Buzz*, p. 86).

Mellow Dude. Calm individual who is able to control his emotions.
1966: "Marijuana, not heroin, is the preferred drug among 'mellow dudes.' " (Sutter, "Righteous Dope Fiend," p. 188).

Mellow Yellow. 1960s hoax. Inside scrapings from banana skins that were baked. Allegedly produced effects akin to marihuana. The hoax originated in Haight-Ashbury and was disseminated by the underground press.
1965: "Mellow Yellow." Song recorded by Donovan.

Mesca. Marihuana.
1958: "He was on mesca, tea, marijuana." (Chandler, *Playback*, p. 126).

Meserole. Thick marihuana cigarette; same as panatella.*

Metabolism. The chemical conversion of a drug to other compounds which can then be more readily eliminated from the body.

Metabolites. Chemical compounds that result from the metabolism of administered drugs. THC has over thirty-five metabolites. The first metabolite produced from THC is called eleven-hydroxy-delta-9-tetrahydrocannabinol (11-OH-THC).

Mex, Mexican. Marihuana.

Mexican Brown, Green, Red. High-potency marihuana from Mexico.
1961: "Royo had left Los Angeles with a kilo of long Mexican green, lately smuggled across the border at Tijuana." (Russell, *Sound*, p. 86).

Mezz. Marihuana cigarette (1930s-1940s). From Milton "Mezz" Mezzrow, jazz clarinetist. Mezzrow sold high-potency marihuana on the streets of Harlem. He was arrested in 1940 for possession and served seventeen months in prison.
1936: "The drug and cigarettes containing it are known as . . . 'mezz.' " (Spencer, "Marihuana," p. 300).
1937: "It now is being called . . . 'mezz.' " (Cooper, *Here's to Crime*, p. 333).
1944: "I had a trey ounce of mezz and that ain't hay." (Marcovitz and Myers, "Marihuana Addict," p. 391).
1946: ". . . the mezz and the mighty mezz, referring, I blush to say, to me and the tea both." (Mezzrow and Wolfe, *Really the Blues*, p. 211).

Mezz Roll. Fat marihuana cigarette (1930s-1940s).
1946: "Mezz roll . . . the kind of fat, well-packed, and clean cigarette I used to roll." (Mezzrow and Wolfe, *Really the Blues*, p. 211).

Mezzony, Mizzony. 1. Money for purchase of marihuana or other drugs.
2. Meeting between buyer and seller of drugs (1930s-1940s).
1936: "Mezzony: about to score a connection." (Maurer, "Argot of Underworld," p. 124).
1942: "Mezzony." (Berrey and Bark, *Thesaurus*, p. 479).

Middling. Acting as a middleman between dealer and buyer.
1976: "Would you be interested in middling it for me?" (Sorfleet, "Dealing," p. 132).

Miggles. *See* Muggles.

Mighty Mezz. Potent marihuana cigarette.

Ming. Marihuana cigarette made of roaches.*

Mitchum, Robert. Film actor. First major movie star to be arrested on marihuana charges (1948). Mitchum was convicted and served a fifty-day sentence, but, in a retrial, the guilty verdict was overturned and he was completely exonerated. The trial was, for many Americans, the first indication that marihuana usage was not confined to the underworld or minority groups.

Moggles. *See* Muggles.

Mohasky. Marihuana.
1943: "Marihuana may be called . . . 'mohasky.' " (*Time*, July 19, p. 54).

Misdemeanor. A criminal offense, less than a felony, the sentence for which may or may not result in incarceration.
1971: "At first you was a 'misdomeanor.' But as the years rolled on you lost your misdo and got meanor and meanor." (Jones and Chilton, *Louis*, p. 116).

Mojo. Any narcotic drug, including marihuana (1930s-1940s).

Moocah, Mootah, Mooter, Mootie, Motta. Marihuana. From the Mexican term *mota; see* appendix.
1926: "Moota." (*New Orleans Morning Tribune*, October 17, p. 1/1).
1931: "In the South amongst the Negros, it is termed 'mooter.' " (Stanley, "Marihuana," p. 253).
1937: "Some people call it . . . 'moocah.' " (Anslinger, "Marihuana," p. 150).
1938: "The drug is known by many different names, such as . . . 'motta,' 'mooter,' . . ." (Yawger, "Marihuana," p. 351).
1938: "A large number of boys of school age buy and smoke 'mootas.' " (Walton, *Marihuana*, p. 30).

Mor a Grifa. Marihuana.
1966: "Mor a Grifa." (Siragusa, *Trail of the Poppy*, p. 232).
1977: "Mor a grifa." (Lentini, *Vice*, p. 139).

Moreau, Jacques-Joseph (de Tours) (1804-1884). French physician who traveled through Arab countries where he became interested in hashish. In 1845 he published *Hashish and Mental Illness*, detailing experiments he conducted on the effects of hashish. Moreau is generally considered to be the physician who introduced Gautier to hashish and who administered hashish to the members of the Club des Haschischins.*

Mu. Marihuana. Shortened version of moocah.*
1936: "The drug and cigarettes containing it are known as . . . 'mu.' "
(Spencer, "Marihuana," p. 300).
1937: "Some people call it 'mu.' " (Anslinger, "Marihuana," p. 150).
1938: "The drug is known by many different names, such as . . .
'mu.' " (Yawger, "Marihuana," p. 351).
1943: "Mu." (*Time*, July 19, p. 54).

Mud. 1. Crude marihuana. 2. Hashish.
1939: "Mud: Hashish." (Housley, *Dictionary*, p. 32).

Muggles. Marihuana cigarettes. Also called miggles, moggles.
1926: "Muggles." (*New Orleans Morning Tribune*, October 1).
1928: "Muggles." Song recorded by Louis Armstrong.
1928: "Add a jot of 'muggles' to the artistic temperament of your
journeyman musician and you've got discord." (*Chicago
Tribune*, July 1, p. 12).
1931: "The muggles habit once firmly established in this country will
never be eradicated." (Fossier, "Marihuana Menace," p. 248).
1931: "It is popularly known amongst the criminal element as
'muggles.' " (Stanley, "Marihuana," p. 255).
1933: ". . . locally designated by such names as . . . 'moota,' 'muggles'
. . ." (Hayes and Bowery, "Marihuana," p. 1087).
1934: "My first experience with a 'muggles' was unfortunately not the
last." (De Lenoir, *Hundredth Man*, p. 220).
1937: "Police in Baltimore were called to investigate the selling of
'muggles' to high-school boys and girls." (Cooper, *Here's to
Crime*, p. 336).
1938: "Guy don't even know a muggles when he sees one." (St. Johns,
"Walking," p. 104).
1949: "Desk clerk's a muggle smoker." (Chandler, *Little Sister*, p.
271).
1951: "Anyone on 'muggles' must become a lawbreaker to a certain
degree." (Lait and Mortimer, *Washington Confidential*, p. 147).
1953: "Muggles." (Burroughs, *Junkie*, p. 18).
1958: "The muggles I mean." (Chandler, *Playback*, p. 104).

Muggle Head. Marihuana user.
1926: "Muggle head." (*New Orleans Morning Tribune*, October 1, p. 1,
col. 2).
1931: "Addicts are commonly termed 'muggle heads.' " (Stanley,
"Marihuana," p. 255).
1949: "Muggle head." (Monteleone, *Criminal Slang*, p. 159).

Muggled Up. Under the influence of marihuana.

1934: "Somebody laughingly remarked that he would give a great deal
to see the Englishman 'muggled up.' " (De Lenoir, *Hundredth
Man*, p. 222).

Mule. 1. Drug smuggler. 2. Marihuana mixed with whiskey.

1974: "If you agree and cocaine or marijuana is later found in the
valise, you have become a 'mule.' " (*High Times*, vol. 1, no. 3,
p. 12).

1977: "The importer may bring in as much as 500 pounds or more
using 'mules' (couriers) to do the actual transporting." (Lentini,
Vice, p. 115).

1955: "Mule." (Braddy, "Narcotic Argot," p. 87).

Munchies. Acute hunger sensation after smoking marihuana.

1971: "Munchies." (Eschholz and Rosa, "Slang," p. 16).

1979: "It's the thing that gives you the munchies." (Goldman,
Grass Roots, p. 38).

1980: "We get the munchies because dope is a stimulant." (Novak,
High Culture, p. 42).

Murder Weed. Marihuana.

1935: "Murder weed." (Pollock, *Underworld Speaks*, p. 20).

Muta. Marihuana. *See also* Mootah.

1946: "He drank quite a lot, but he was a strict Catholic and was
dead against the muta." (Mezzrow and Wolfe, *Really the Blues*,
p. 150).

1971: "He said, 'Louis, this muta (one of the names the Fays used)
. . .' " (Jones and Chilton, *Louis*, p. 115).

N

Nabilone. Drug synthesized by Eli Lilly Co. It has many of the same
effects as THC.

Nabs. Police.

Nail. Marihuana cigarette.

Narc, Narco. 1. Federal narcotics officer. 2. Undercover agent who
associates with drug users to gather evidence, which later will be used
against them.

1960: "With the narcos sending in bearded, poetry-writing undercover men to make the scene and raid the tea-parties." (Chiardi, *Saturday Review*, p. 12).

1964: "Four by narcos." (Harris, *Junkie Priest*, p. 2).

1967: ". . . just out of the clutches of the local narcos." (Ric, *Esquire*, September, p. 101).

Narcotic. Medically, a substance that induces sleep (narcosis). Generally applied to drugs that also cause a stupor and relieve pain. Legally, a term given to any habit-forming drug, for example, heroin, morphine. The term is incorrectly applied to marihuana and cocaine.

Narcotic Control Act (1956). Law increasing penalties for marihuana possession or sale. Possession of any amount carried a minimum two-year sentence for the first offense, a five-year sentence for the second offense, and ten-years for the third and all subsequent sentences. The fine for all offenses was $20,000. Sale carried a minimum five-year sentence for the first offense and ten years for the second and all subsequent convictions. Probation and parole were denied for any but first-possession offenders.

National Commission on Marihuana and Drug Abuse. *See* Shafer Commission.

Nepalese Hash. Potent hashish originating in Nepal.

Nepalese Temple Balls, Nepalese Temple Hash. Balls of hashish used in Hindu religious ceremonies. Now imported for profane use. *See also* Temple Balls.

1971: "Nepalese Temple Balls." (*Marihuana Review*, vol. 1, no. 8, p. 24).

1974: "Nepalese hashish hand-rubbed fingers and balls. . ." (*High Times*, vol. 1, no. 2, p. 39).

Nepenthes. Drug mentioned by poet Homer in his *Odyssey* (4: 219-32); literally "against sorrow." Although not specifically identified, occasionally argued that it was marihuana, although opium is also a common suggestion.

Neurosine. Drug preparation containing marihuana. Sold during 1930s.

New York White. *See* Manhattan Silver.

Nickel Bag. Five-dollar packet of marihuana.

1967: "A nickel bag—five dollars' worth—should be a fifth of an ounce." (Ric, *Esquire*, September, p. 191).

NIDA. National Institute on Drug Abuse. Created in 1073, this Federal agency was responsible for providing means for prevention, control, and treatment of drug abuse. It was also responsible for issuing reports to Congress summarizing research regarding marihuana.

NIMH. National Institute of Mental Health.

Noble Weed. Marihuana.
1970: "Noble weed." (Gardner, "Slang," p. 21).

Nod. Stupor; drowsy sleep produced by drugs.
1968: "If he wants to nod he gets marihuana soaked in opium." (Bloomquist, *Marihuana*, p. 190).

Nodding. Stuporous.
1955. "So I sit here, and I'm nodding." (Braddy, "Anonymous Verses," p. 132).

NORML. National Organization for the Reform of Marihuana Laws. Washington, D.C. based national lobbying group advocating more lenient marihuana laws at federal and state levels.

Nose Burner. Butt of marihuana cigarette. *See also* Roach.

Nose Warmer. *See* nose burner.

"Notch Number One." Western starring Ben Wilson; first (1925) movie to feature marihuana as a plot device.

Number. Marihuana cigarette.
1963: "You smoke this number while I go and call John." (University of California, *Folklore*, p. 267).
1969: ". . . the grass cigarette, or joint, stick, number, Jay, or reefer." (Margolis and Clorfene, *Grass*, p. 99).
1970: "Number." (Brennan, *Drugs*, p. 79).

O

O. Ounce of marihuana. *See also* O.Z.
1960: "O." (De Mexico, *Marijuana Girl*, p. 155).

Oaxacan. Potent marihuana from the Mexican state of Oaxacan.
1976: "How is someone from Colby, Kansas, supposed to know with any certainty his pot is Oaxacan." (*Marijuana Monthly*, March, p. 58).

O.D. Overdose. Administration of a quantity of drug greater than that normally used. Generally used in reference to narcotic dose that results in death. Sometimes used to indicate drug dose resulting in unpleasant reaction.

ODALE. Office of Drug Abuse Law Enforcement. Established in 1972, the agency was responsible for development and enforcement of federal drug abuse laws. It was abolished in 1973.

Ohio Bag. Baggie containing 100 g of marihuana—the quantity that qualifies as the amount required for a simple possession fine under Ohio's decriminalization law.

Oil. Hash oil.*

Oiler. Hash oil* user.

O.J. Opium joint. Marihuana cigarette dipped in liquid opium. It was popular in Vietnam. *See* Atom Bomb, Candy a Joint.
1970: ". . . in the evening would wind up the day either smoking 'O.J.'s,' marihuana dipped in liquid opium . . ." (Kaplan, "*Marihuana,*" p. 261).
1972: "An 'OJ'—GI style marihuana joint . . ." (Westin and Shaffer, *Heroes*, p. 19).

Old Man of the Mountain. *See* Assassins.

On. High; under the influence of marihuana. *See also* Turn on, Turned on.
1967: "You on, man?" (Thomas, *Mean Streets*, p. 121).

On the nod. *See* Nod.

One, The. Hash oil.* Alcoholic extract of marihuana. Dark, viscous liquid. Commercially available in the United States in 1970. Succeeded in 1971 by Son of One.*
1971: " 'The one' is the first time anything close to real THC has hit the streets." (*Marihuana Review*, vol. 1, no. 8, p. 23).
1977: "The one was around for only a year or so." (*High Times*, February, p. 6).

One-toke Weed. Marihuana so potent only a few inhalations are needed to get high. *See also* Toke.

Operation Intercept. U.S. attempt to shut off the flow of marihuana from Mexico in 1969. The project was abandoned twenty days after initiation, after protests from the Mexican government and American citizens who were subjected to searches and long traffic jams at border.

This operation effectively cut off the supply but it led to imports from other countries and possible experimentation with "harder," more available drugs.

Opiated Hash. Hashish to which opium has been added.

Oregon Decriminalization Bill. First (1973) state law decriminalizing marihuana from a felony to a $100 civil misdemeanor.

O'Shaughnessy, Dr. William B. Irish physician who was professor of chemistry at the Medical College of Calcutta during the mid-1800s. O'Shaughnessy conducted studies of cannabis as a drug to treat rheumatism, tetanus, epilepsy, cholera, and rabies. Although it did not cure any of these diseases, he found that patients gained considerable relief. Largely through publication of his experiments, Western doctors became acquainted with and eager to try cannabis as a medicine in their own practices.

Out. No longer high on marihuana.
1938: "The experienced smoker is able to go 'in' and 'out' at will." (Yawger, "Marihuana," p. 355).

Out of sight. Excellent, superior, first rate.

O.Z. Ounce of marihuana or any other drug.
1953: "It had been something in his mind that two O.Z.'s of ripe Pachuto pot had brought out." (Holmes, *Horn*, p. 224).
1960: "OZ." (De Mexico, *Marijuana Girl*, p. 155).

P

P.R. *See* Panama Red.

Pack (of Rockets, of Rocks). Package of marihuana cigarettes.
1949: "Pack of rocks." (Monteleone, *Criminal Slang*, p. 170).

Pad. 1. Place where drugs such as marihuana are used. 2. Room, apartment, sleeping quarters.
1938: "It is in Harlem, where the price is generally fifteen cents and two for a quarter that the pads (reefer smoking dens) are thickest." (*Fortune*, July, p. 60).
1955: *"Twas the night before Christmas*
And all through the pad

Reefers and cocaine
Was all that we had . . ."
(Braddy, "Anonymous Verses," p. 131).

Pakistani Hash. Potent hashish originating in Pakistan.
1972: "After Pakistan hash, it's impossible to get a real stone on the
grass around here." (Hall, *Heads*, p. 66).

Panama Canal Zone Military Inquiry (1916-1929). First official U.S.
inquiry into the effects of marihuana. The investigation centered on
marihuana usage by American soldiers serving in the Panama Canal
Zone. Despite belief by top army command that marihuana was harmful, the boards of inquiry repeatedly found no evidence to substantiate
this belief.

The inquiry also contained the first officially conducted labora-
tory experiments on the effects of marihuana on human subjects.

Panama Gold. Potent marihuana from Panama; gold in color.
1968: "Panama Gold." (Gross, *Flower People*, p. 176).

Panama Red. Potent marihuana from Panama; red in color.
1967: "Perhaps someone will have some Acapulco Gold or Panama
Red." (Rosevear, *Pot*, p. 32).
1967: "Other prime grass is Panama Red." (*Newsweek*, July 24, p. 48).
1968: " 'Acapulco gold' and 'Panama red' are reputedly especially
potent." (Goode, *Marihuana*, p. 2).
1968: "Because of this 'Acapulco Gold' and 'Panama Red' have become very popular." (Bloomquist, *Marihuana*, p. 190).
1979: ". . . somebody's extraspecial super-great Panama Red . . ."
(Goldman, *Grass Roots*, p. 27).

Panatella. 1. Thickly rolled marihuana cigarette. Originally an expensive cigar. 2. Potent marihuana, sold for a quarter per cigarette in
1940s.
1944: "The 'panatella' cigarette, occasionally referred to as meserole,
is considered more potent than 'sass-fras' and usually retails for
approximately 25 cents each." (*La Guardia Report*, p. 9).
1946: "They rolled it in a different sized paper, about half an inch
longer than mine and much thinner, and they called their product
'panatella.' " (Mezzrow and Wolfe, *Really the Blues*, p. 224).
1956: "Jimmy's got the best panatella you ever smoked." (Holiday,
Lady, p. 53).
1959: "Panatella." Song recorded by Woody Herman.

Pancho Villa. Mexican revolutionary of early twentieth century who raided American towns across the Rio Grande. His followers were said to have been marihuana users, thus contributing to the negative attitude to the drug in the Southwest. *See also* Cucaracha.

Pantagruelion. Word used by French writer Francois Rabelais to refer to cannabis.

Papers. Cigarette papers used to make marihuana cigarettes.

Paranoia. Condition bordering on psychosis characterized by extreme suspiciousness of being watched; fear of being arrested.
1969: "Pushers, with good reason, are more paranoid about the police than anything else." (Geller and Boas, *Drug Beat*, p. 68).

Paraquat. Herbicide used by Mexican government beginning in 1975 to eradicate marihuana fields.

Park Lane No. 2s. Marihuana from Cambodia; term used by Americans in Vietnam.
1970: "In Saigon, a package of 20 cigarettes—often the Vietnamese filter tip brand called Parklane—containing marijuana . . ." (*New York Times*, March 22, p. 38).
1971: "Few careermen . . . ever develop a sustained taste for Pleiku Pink, Bleu de Hue, Cambodian made Park Lane No. 2s, and the myriad of other varieties of marihuana that have become freely available in South Vietnam." (*Time*, March 1, p. 15).
1980: "Prerolled joints were sold under the name 'Park Lanes.' " (Novak, *High Culture*, p. 169).

Pato de gayina. Literally "feet of chicken." Form of sinsemilla.* So called because of shape of pod.
1970: "Pato de gayina." (Brennan, *Drugs*, p. 80).

Personal Hash. Hashish sold only to other dealers for personal use; very potent.

Phantastica. Drugs producing altered perceptions in which the user is aware of what he is experiencing and can remember what has been experienced, for example, peyote, LSD.

Phenotype. Visible characteristics of genetic inheritance.

Phenotypic ratio. Method of classifying different variants of marihuana according to ratio of three main cannabinoids*:

$$\text{Phenotypic ratio} = \frac{\%\text{Delta-9-THC} + \%\text{CBN}}{\%\text{CBD}}$$

The higher the ratio, the higher the psychoactive potential of a plant.

Pick up. Smoke marihuana.
1946: "Where can I pick up?" (Charen and Perelman, "Marihuana Addicts," p. 678).

Pick up smoking. Sharing a marihuana cigarette.

Piece. Ounce of marihuana.

Pig. Police officer.

Pig Rap. Discussion among drug users about police harassment.

Pin. Thin marihuana cigarette.
1967: ". . . handmade cigarettes, called joints, reefers, sticks, pins, things, and so on." (Rosevear, *Pot*, p. 64).
1969: "Very thin joints are called Very Thin Joints (although very thin people call them Pins)." (Margolis and Clorfene, *Grass*, p. 102).

Pinner. *See* Pin.

Placebo. Inert material.

Plant. 1. To place marihuana in someone's property that will later be found and used as evidence of possession. 2. An informant.

Played. Completely smoked.

Pleiku Pink. Marihuana. Term used by American soldiers in Vietnam. *See also* Park Lane No. 2s.

Pod. Marihuana.
1952: "You can smoke all the pod you want, but keep away from the junkies." (Mandell, *Flee the Angry Strangers*, p. 30).
1952: "So Dianne smoked jive, pod, and tea." (*New York Times*, April 19, p. 25).
1955: "I got no eyes for turning on with pod." (White, "Wayne University," p. 304).
1959: "Talks about 'pod' . . . " (Burroughs, *Naked Lunch*, p. 2).

Poke. Inhalation of marihuana smoke or opium. *See also* Toat, Toke.
1955: "I took a few pokes/ And Man I got stoned." (Braddy, "Anonymous Verses," p. 136).
1956: "Sure you don't want a poke?" (Duke, *Sideman*, p. 274).
1965: "I held it like he did and took a poke just the way he did." (Becker, *Outsiders*, p. 48).

Poking. Smoking marihuana.

Popo Oro. Potent marihuana from Mexico.

Popped. Arrested.
1974: ". . . popped with 10 pounds of dope after his common-law wife
     tipped off police." (*High Times*, vol. 1, no. 1, p. 32).

Pot. Marihuana. Most popular term for marihuana in the 1950s. Pot
has various suggested origins. Maurer ("Argot of Underworld," p. 189)
contended it came from a Portuguese word, *potaguaya*, which he defined as marihuana pods after the leaves had been removed. He subsequently ("Marihuana Addicts," p. 572) refined this definition: "The
ripe female flowering tops are stripped of their leaves and are then
known to dealers and addicts as potiguaya." This derivation has
largely been followed by many writers although Maurer himself
abandoned it (*Narcotics*, p. 380), claiming that the term originated
from the Mexican-Spanish term *potacion de guaya*, meaning "drink of
grief."

Both Portuguese and Mexican origins are probably incorrect. Since
there is no input from either the Portuguese language or culture on
marihuana usage in the United States, the first suggestion is highly unlikely. The second suggestion, while possible, is also highly unlikely because of the lateness of the appearance of the term "pot." Had pot
originated from the Mexican it would have appeared during the 1920s
or 1930s, along with words such as *griefa* and *muta*, which subsequently gave way to reefer and mooter, respectively.

Gold *(Jazz Lexicon)* suggests that the term originated from the
fact that marihuana was grown in flower pots during the 1940s. Users
simply referred to the plant by way of its container. This theory has
nothing to support it. Only in the 1960s and 1970s was marihuana
raised in private homes in flower pots. Previous to that, it was either
imported or taken from vacant lots where it grew wild.

Dr. Michael Aldrich, curator of the Fitzhugh Ludlow Library (San
Francisco), relays another theory that traces the word to the practice
of making tea from marihuana. Because marihuana was occasionally
brewed in a teapot, pot became a shortened way of referring to the
drug. While tea was and still is a common term for marihuana, relatively little marihuana was, or is, consumed as tea in the United States.
The reason marihuana was called tea is more likely due to its appearance.

Yet another possibility, which is merely speculative, is that the term
is derived from another term, "pod," which came into the language at
about the same time as pot. Pod referred to the flowering marihuana
pod. In 1952, Mandell (*Flee the Angry Strangers*, p. 30) touches on
this possibility:

" 'Pod, Dincher; don't say pot.'
'What's the diff? You wanna get on?'
'Don't say pot, Dinch. It's the intellectuals from college and all who come
on that way. They want to get their hip-cards punched. Say pod, Dincher.' "

The earliest appearance for either term is 1951.

1951: ". . . progression from sneaky pete to pot to horse to banging."
(*New York Times*, June 14, p. 22/2).

1951: "I heard and saw guys who skin pop, snut, smoke pot, banging
and shoot up the main vein . . ." (*Life*, June 25, p. 21/1).

1952: "I got some pot stashed away by the subway." (Mandell, *Flee
the Angry Strangers*, p. 30).

1953: "Benny times, pot times, junk times, mad times." (Holmes,
Horn, p. 199).

1955: " 'You was smoking pot and getting wild, so they kicked your
ass out of there before the cops came up.' " (Ellson, *Rock*, p.
36).

1956: "He must be cutting off her supply of heroin and pot." (Trujillo,
I Love You, p. 11).

1956: "Those dope stories—all about how you go around killing old
ladies when you smoke a pot." (Longstreet, *Real Jazz*, p. 146).

1957: "Goldie twittered and asked if he would like some pot." (Selby,
Last Exit, p. 39).

1959: "Every user I know calls it pot." (Lipton, *Holy Barbarians*,
p. 21).

1960: "She had smoked pot for years but her attitude toward heroin
was rigid." (Trocchi, *Cain's Book*, p. 18).

Pot Head. Frequent marihuana user.

1961: "Gil is a somewhat pothead junkie." (Hughes, *Fantastic Lodge*,
p. 145).

1966: "The 'pot heads,' for example, are 'ultra cool', use no other
drugs, and often prefer soda-pop to liquor." (Sutton, "Righteous
Dope Fiend," p. 191).

1967: "Pot heads who buy kilos must have connections." (Simmons,
Marihuana, p. 84).

1967: "Most of these potheads are college students." (*Look*, August
18, p. 12).

1980: "They might think I was a pothead." (Novak, *High Culture*,
p. 212).

Pot Likker, Liquor. Tea brewed with marihuana.

1967: "It is ubiquitous and easily grown, can be smoked in 'joints' (cigarettes), baked into cookies or brewed in tea ('pot likker').'' (*Time*, July 7, p. 21).

1977: "Pot likker." (Lentini, *Vice*, p. 141).

Pot Lush. Chronic marihuana user.

1969: "The archaic antiestablishment attitude of these 'pot lushes' . . .'' (*Time*, July 25, p. 65).

Pot out. Smoke marihuana.

1970: "Pot out." (Gardner, *Current Slang*, vol. 4, no. 2, p. 8).

Pot Party. Gathering of people to smoke marihuana.

1965: ". . . an occasional but much headlined arrest of a pot party where college students are present." (*New York Post*, December 3, p. 45/3).

1967: "There had been no advance notice that this would be a pot party." (Simmons, *Marihuana*, p. 28).

1969: "Their pot parties represent a sort of collective, community narcissism." (*Time*, July 25, p. 65).

Potency. Strength of action. The quantity of drug producing a particular response. The smaller the amount, the greater the potency; for example, hashish is more potent than marihuana. The higher up the marihuana plant that material is taken, the more potent; for example, flowers are more potent than leaves. The potency of the plant itself is determined by genetic factors. THC is about three times more potent when smoked compared to when it is eaten.

Potentiation. Combined effect of two or more drugs such that the combination produces a greater effect than either alone. *See* A Bomb, Candy a Joint.

Potted. Under the influence of marihuana.

1955: "Potted." (Trujillo, *I Love You*, p. 138).

Pound Action. Buying a pound of marihuana.

1967: "When a pound is considered, the term is naturally called 'pound action.' '' (Rosevear, *Pot*, p. 28).

Powder. Marihuana; hashish.

1954: ". . . weed, slag, powder, charge or gear." (Bevan, *Everybody's*, June 12, p. 13).

Power Hit. Inhaling smoke from a marihuana cigarette and then blowing it into another smoker's mouth as he inhales.

1970: "Power hit." (Brennan, *Drugs*, p. 82).

1974: "The first person blows a jet-stream of pure smoke into the mouth of the recipient. This is also known as a power hit." (Isyurhash and Rusoff, *Gourmet*, p. 54).

President Johnson's Commission on Law Enforcement and Administration of Justice. Commission appointed by President Johnson in 1967 to study drug laws. Commission urged distinction between narcotics and marihuana.

President Kennedy's Ad Hoc Panel on Drug Abuse. Panel appointed by President Kennedy in 1962 to study the drug abuse problem in the U.S. The panel dismissed the alleged connection between marihuana and sexual abuse as unfounded. It also claimed that dangers associated with marihuana were exaggerated and said current penalties imposed on occasional users or possessors were in "poor social perspective."

President's Advisory Commission on Narcotics and Drug Abuse. *See* Prettyman Commission.

Prettyman Commission. Commission appointed in 1963 by President Kennedy to review the drug problem in the U.S. The commission recommended that minimum mandatory sentences as prescribed by the Boggs Act be reconsidered; the transfer of the Bureau of Narcotics from the treasury department to the Department of Health, Education, and Welfare; and increased money be allocated for research into the effects of marihuana. It also recommended that marihuana be distinguished from narcotics.

Primo. First-rate; excellent.
1971: "Primo sells for $5 a pound in Afghanistan." (Coyote Man, *Buzz*, p. 5).
1974: "Primo grass consists of the flowering tops of matured and cured plants." (Isyurhash and Rusoff, *Gourmet*, p. 4).
1975: ". . . the fabled Afghani primo is not as available . . ." (*High Times*, October, p. 43).
1979: "First quality, Primo hashish is considered to be the most powerful and most priceless." (Cherniak, *Hashish*, p. 25).

Psychedelic. Mind expanding. Term invented by Humphrey Osmond in correspondence with Aldous Huxley in 1956. From Greek *psyche* (soul) and *delos* (visible).

Psychoactive. Any drug that acts on the mind.

Psychodysleptic. Mind distorting.

Psycholytic. Mind loosening.

Psychosis. Severe mental disturbance in which individual loses touch with reality and may experience hallucinations* or delusions.

Psychotomimetic. A substance capable of initiating activity in the brain.

Psychotropic. *See* psychoactive.*

Pull. Deep inhalation of smoke from a marihuana cigarette.

Punk. Low-potency marihuana.

Punta Roja. Literally "red point." Potent marihuana from Colombia.
1978: "A punta roja high can be very trippy and meditative." (*High Times*, July, p. 39).

Pure Food and Drug Act (1906). U.S. law requiring all patent medicines shipped across state lines to list their ingredients if they contained more than a specified amount of certain drugs, including cannabis.

Pusher. Drug seller. Usually in reference to narcotics, whereas dealer* is a term used to refer to a marihuana seller. Sometimes also used to refer to a marihuana seller.
1938: "I know all the big pushers (peddlers) in the state." (Rowell, *David Dare*, p. 14).
1958: "He was on the weed. I pretended to be a pusher." (Chandler, *Playback*, p. 134).
1962: "Pushing is disgusting, there's no character in it. And besides, it's a Federal rap." (Pritchie, *Savage Kick*, p. 126).

Put on the hempen collar. To be hanged. *See also* Hemp.

Q

Quarter Bag. One ounce of marihuana.

Quarter Moon. Hashish.

Quarter Ounce. One-fifth of an ounce of marihuana.
1976: "The occasional dealer, who deals only for 'free smoke,' buys an ounce of hashish for $95 or $100, and divides it into five equal parts which are then sold as 'quarter ounces.' " (Sorfleet, "Dealing," p. 130).

R

Ragweed. Marihuana.
1972: "Ragweed." (Smith and Gray, *It's So Good*, p. 205).

Railroad Weed. Marihuana.

Randall, Robert. First American since 1937 legally permitted to smoke marihuana. Usage was allowed on the grounds that marihuana lessened the effects of his glaucoma and that without it he would become blind. Official recognition that marihuana has therapeutic value undermines Comprehensive Drug Abuse Prevention and Control Act of 1970, which sanctioned antimarihuana laws on grounds that marihuana has no therapeutic value. *See also* Controlled Substance Act.

Rangoon. Marihuana.
1968: "Rangoon." (Dawtry, *Drug Abuse*, p. 94).

Rap. Talk, conversation.
1974: "A dealer's rap about grades of grass can become confusing."
    (*High Times*, vol. 1, no. 1, p. 8).

Rastafarians. Black Jamaican religious cult that regarded Haile Selasse, whose name was Ras Tafari before becoming emperor of Ethiopia, as the living god. The Rastafarians call themselves black Hebrews and Lions of Judah and regard themselves as one of the ten lost tribes of Israel. They take the biblical verse, "Thou shall eat the herb of the field," as a reference to marihuana (ganja) and take it in their tea or smoke it as a religious sacrament.

Rat. An informer; to inform.

Recreational Drug. Drug regarded as benign and controllable; "soft" drug,* for example, marihuana, in contrast to "hard" drug, for example, heroin.

Red. Marihuana, short for Panama Red.*

Red Dirt Marihuana. Uncultivated, wild marihuana.
1960: "Red Dirt Marihuana." Title of short story by T. Southern,
    Esquire, p. 61).

Red Gunyon. Powdered marihuana seed pods smoked in a water pipe.

Red Leb(anese). Potent hashish originating in Lebanon; reddish in color.

Red Oil. Hash oil.*

Reefer. Marihuana cigarette. Most common word for marihuana in the 1930s. The term possibly derived from Mexican *grifa*, or *grifo*, which originally meant someone intoxicated. Owing to Mexican tendency to elide the g at the beginning of a word, *grifa* became *rifa*. When picked up by Americans, *rifa*, became *reefa*, and then reefer.

1931: "That Funny Reefer Man." Song recorded by Don Redman.

1936: "The drug and cigarettes containing it are known as . . . reefers." (Spencer, "Marihuana," p. 300).

1937: "Some people call it . . . 'reefers.' " (Anslinger, "Marihuana," p. 150).

1937: "The use of 'reefers' has grown so swiftly that it has all but enveloped America." (Cooper, *Here's to Crime*, p. 337).

1938: "The reefers are hand made." (Berger, *New Yorker*, March 12, p. 48).

1938: "After smoking a reefer, she was able to dance long without fatigue." (Yawger, "Marihuana," p. 356).

1941: "It wasn't just a private hallucination of his own brought on by the reefers." (Irish, *Marihuana*, p. 71).

1945: "I'm gonna set right down and roll myself a reefer." (Saxon, *Gumbo*, p. 462).

1950: " 'Smoking a reefer,' Rodina laughed, 'You know—dope.' " (Smith, *Anger*, p. 201).

1965: "He'd never smoked pot until I gave him a reefer one night." (Brown, *Manchild*, p. 161).

1968: "I smoked reefer for five straight years before I ever knew what heroin was." (Heard, *Howard Street*, p. 203).

1969: "I took a deep pull on the stick of reefer." (Iceberg Slim, *Pimp*, p. 84).

1971: "Jimmy lit a reefer." (Woodley, *Dealer*, p. 193).

1974: "A whole boatload of reefer . . ." (*High Times*, vol. 1, no. 3, p. 5).

Reefer Hound. Marihuana smoker.

1948: "Reefer hound." (Gottschalk and Cowdry, *Language*, p. 12).

"Reefer Madness." 1938 movie about alleged evils of marihuana. Now regarded as a cult film.

Reefer Man. Marihuana seller.

1931: "Reefer Man." Song recorded by Don Redman.

1935: "A 'reefer man' is a peddler who bootlegs these cigarettes." (Calloway, *His Hi De Highness*, p. 36).

Reefing Man. Marihuana user.

1936: "Reefing man." (Maurer, "Argot of Underworld," p. 125).

1949: "Reefing man." (Monteleone, *Criminal Slang*, p. 192).

Reverse Tolerance. Increased sensitivity to a drug as a result of previous usage. Opposite of tolerance.*

Righteous. Unadulterated, pure, honest, good, pleasurable. *See also* Righteous Bush, Righteous Dealer.

1938: "I want to pickle some of that righteous junk." (Walton, *Marihuana*, p. 195).

1976: "Dealers who buy from me look forward eagerly to my male plants, because they know the smoke will be righteous." (*High Times*, November, p. 102).

Righteous Bush. Marihuana.

1946: ". . . the hard-cuttin' mezz and the righteous bush." (Mezzrow and Wolfe, *Really the Blues*, p. 211).

1959: "Righteous Bush." (Schmidt, *Narcotics*, p. 69).

Righteous Dealer. Honest marihuana seller.

1974: "The righteous dealer is a rare and wonderful breed." (Isyurhash and Rusoff, *Gourmet*, p. 36).

Rip off. To cheat or steal.

1974: "Soon, hopefully, rip-offs, busts and burns will be a thing of the past." (Isyurhash and Rusoff, *Gourmet*, p. 36).

Ripped. Very intoxicated.

Rizla. Brand of marihuana cigarette paper.

1969: "Friends also suggested a Rizla rolling machine." (*Time*, September 26, p. 73).

1974: "In my experience, the standard brands such as zig zag or rizla are the best." (Isyurhash and Rusoff, *Gourmet*, p. 52).

Roach. Marihuana cigarette butt. So-called because the butt has the appearance of a roach to some smokers.

1946: "Roaches were passed round and round." (Mezzrow and Wolfe, *Really the Blues*, p. 206).

1952: ". . . reached into a crate for a last night's roach." (Mandell, *Flee the Angry Strangers*, p. 177).

1952: "There may be a roach around here somewhere." (Burroughs, *Junkie*, p. 33).

1956: "There's more power when it's down to the roach." (Hunter, *Second Ending*, p. 247).

1956: ". . . the marihuana cigarette which he smokes down to the roach, the smallest butt in the world." (Longstreet, *Real Jazz*, p. 144).

1957: "She sucked the joint down to an 1/8th of an inch then dropped the roach into her mouth." (Selby, *Last Exit*, p. 38).

1968: ". . . burnt to a little bit of a roach." (Thomas, *Mean Streets*, p. 65).

1969: "I lit it and sucked it into a 'roach.' " (Iceberg Slim, *Pimp*, p. 152).

Roach Bender. Marihuana user.

1942: "Roach bender." (Berrey and Bark, *Thesaurus*, p. 476).

1967: "He may also be called a 'roach bender,' 'tea man,' 'weed hound' . . ." (Bloomquist, *Marihuana*, p. 48).

Roach Clip. Device to hold the remaining tip of a marihuana cigarette so that it can be smoked to the very end. *See also* Bridge, Jefferson Airplane.

1969: "Another important purchase was a roach clip." (*Time*, September 26, p. 73).

1969: "The best method is to purchase a roach holder or roach clip." (Margolis and Clorfene, *Grass*, p. 108).

1970: "They were pelted by the hail of roach clips." (Sanders, *Shards*, p. 95).

1980: "Save your roach-clips, they'll soon become collectors' items." (Novak, *High Culture*, p. 234).

Rock Out. To fall asleep from too much marihuana.

1972: "Rock out." (Folb, *Black Argot*, p. 114).

Rocket. Marihuana.

1942: "Rocket." (Berrey and Bark, *Thesaurus*, p. 474).

1968: "It is referred to as a 'reefer,' 'rocket,' 'stick,' 'joint,' or 'weed.' " (Bloomquist, *Marihuana*, p. 48).

Roll (up). To make a marihuana cigarette.

1936: "I pawned my shoes for one dollar and bought a bag of dried leaves to roll my own." (Spencer, "Marihuana," p. 302).

1965: "I had to show him how to roll pot." (Brown, *Manchild*, p. 162).

1967: "Red rolled two more sticks." (Chaplin, *Grass*, p. 133).

Rolling Buzz. Mild intoxication experienced some time after smoking marihuana. *See also* Buzz.

1966: "Gnosos had stopped smoking anything but was still high enough for a rolling buzz." (Farina, *Been Down So Long*, p. 12).

Rolling Machine. Device for rolling marihuana cigarettes. *See* Roll.

Rolling Paper. Double-width cigarette paper used primarily for making marihuana cigarettes. Currently there are 300 to 400 different brands available, ranging in price from ten cents to a dollar a package. Papers are flavored, for example, strawberry, banana, grape; are made from different kinds of material, for example, wheat, rice; and contain various printed material on them, for example, cartoons. *See* Bambu, E-Z Wider, Rizla.

Root. Marihuana cigarette.
1965: "The drug's traditional association with sex may be responsible for the marihuana cigarette's being called a 'joint' and a 'root.' " (Winick, "Marihuana," p. 233).

Rope. Marihuana. So called because marihuana smoke smells like burnt rope or because most rope was initially made from the fibers of the marihuana plant. *See* Hemp.
1968: "Rope." (Dawtry, *Drug Abuse*, p. 94).
1974: "I think he smokes rope." (Schiano, *Solo*, p. 11).

Rosa Maria. Marihuana.

Rough Stuff. Uncleaned marihuana.

Rowell, Earle Albert. Antimarihuana crusader of 1930s. In 1938, Rowell was arrested for possession of an opium pipe and a small amount of narcotics he used in his lectures. Smear tactics were used against him by the Federal Narcotics Bureau because of his criticism of the bureau. He is the author of the antimarihuana polemic *On the Trail of Marihuana: The Weed of Madness* (1939).

Run. Prolonged period of drug use. More often used in reference to drugs such as amphetamines than marihuana.

Runner. Delivery man for drug seller.

Running Amok. *See* Amok.

Rush. Intense euphoric reaction from drug use. Initially used in reference to effects of narcotics injection.
1971: "Rush: a sudden feeling of elatedness derived from the use of marihuana." (*Current Slang*, vol. 5, no. 5, p. 19).
1974: "Smoking light hash or grass after the initial rush . . ." (Isyurhash and Rusoff, *Gourmet*, p. 17).
1976: "One gets a rush after just one hit, and the only way to finish a Mombasa joint is to smoke it like a cigarette." (*High Times*, November, p. 86).

S

Sagebrush Whacker. Marihuana user.
1959: "Sagebrush whacker." (Schmidt, *Narcotics*, p. 162).

Salt and Pepper. Weak marihuana; marihuana adulterated with oregano.
1959: "Salt and pepper." (Murtagh and Harris, *Who Live in Shadows*,
    p. 205).

Sam. Federal narcotics officer; from "Uncle Sam."

Santa Maria Gold. Potent marihuana from Colombia; gold in color.

Santa Maria Red. Potent marihuana from Colombia; red in color.

Sass-fras. Weak marihuana cigarette made from marihuana grown in
the United States during the 1940s.
1944: "The cheapest brand is known as 'sass-fras,' and retails for approx-
    imately three for 50 cents." (*La Guardia Report*, p. 9).

Sativa. Marihuana, from *Cannabis sativa*, the botanical name for the
marihuana plant.

Sausage. Marihuana.
1968: "Sausage." (Dawtry, *Drug Abuse*, p 94).

Scarf. *See* Scroff.

Scene. Place where something is happening, for example, where marihuana is being used.
1957: "I make it my business to stay in the scene." (Braddy, "Anon-
    ymous Verses," p. 137).

Score. Locate and buy marihuana or any other drug.
1936: "Score." (Maurer, "Argot of Underworld," p. 125).
1974: "Whenever it becomes necessary to score some grass . . ."
    (*High Times*, vol. 1, no. 1, p. 8).
1974: "Scoring dope can be a tremendously exciting experience."
    (Isyurhash and Rusoff, *Gourmet*, p. 35).
1979: "He 'scores' on the school playground." (Goldman, *Grass Roots*,
    p. 10).

Scroff, Scarf. To swallow, for example, to scarf or scroff a marihuana
joint to avoid arrest.
1938: "Scroff." (Maurer, "Argot of Underworld," p. 180).

Sealing Wax. 1. Crude opium. 2. Hashish.
1939: "Sealing wax: hashish." (Housley, *Dictionary*, p. 44).

Seed. Marihuana cigarette butt.

Send. To smoke marihuana.
1936: "To 'send' is to produce the effects caused by smoking."
(Spencer, "Marihuana," p. 300).
1938: "When he reaches a stage of full contentment his body is
'sent.' " (Berger, *New Yorker*, March 12, p. 47).
1946: "Smoking is known as viping or sending." (Maurer, "Marihuana
Addicts," p. 572).

Send up smoke rings. Smoke marihuana.
1959: "Send up smoke rings." (Schmidt, *Narcotics*, p. 164).

Sess. *See* Sinsemilla.

Sessile gland. Gland in marihuana leaf that stores resin containing THC*
produced by trichomes.*

Set. Expectations that affect reaction to drugs. Important only for very
low doses.

Setting. Situation in which drug is taken. Can affect drug reaction
especially for low doses of drugs.

Seven-foot step. Slow, gliding gait of person under the influence of
marihuana.

Shafer Commission. National Commission on Marihuana and Drug
Abuse headed by Chairman Raymond P. Shafer. The commission was
appointed by President Nixon as part of the Comprehensive Drug
Abuse Prevention and Control Act of 1970 (Section 601 of Public
Law 91-513). The commission issued two reports: *Marihuana: Signal
of Misunderstanding* (1972) and *Drug Use in America: Problem in
Perspective* (1973).

The commission recognized widespread use in America and recommended possession no longer be treated as a criminal offense but
considered that sale and distribution of marihuana for profit remain
felonies.

Shake. Resinous material that falls to bottom of sack during transit.
1979: "The next item on the menu is Colombian shake." (Goldman,
Grass Roots, p. 27).

Shishi. Hashish.

Shit. 1. Marihuana. 2. Narcotics.
1946: "Shit." (Charen and Perelman, "Marihuana Addicts," p. 678).

1968: "It certainly was interesting-looking shit." (Farina, *Been Down So Long*, p. 91).

1972: "We lay down our sleeping bags and smoke shit." (Lubin, *Hippies*, p. 127).

1979: "This shit cost me five-fifty." (Goldman, *Grass Roots*, p. 24).

Shlook. Puff of marihuana smoke.

Short. 1. Loosely packed marihuana. 2. Quantity of marihuana that is less than bargained for.

1967: "There are shorts and longs, meaning marihuana is poured into the can for the short, or is packed tightly into the can for the long." (Rosevear, *Pot*, p. 28).

1968: "Cans are of two sizes, short (loosely packed) and long (tightly packed)." (Bloomquist, *Marihuana*, p. 54).

Shotgun. *See* Carburetor.

1977: ". . . gives you a 'shotgun' without sticking a number in your mouth." (*High Times*, April, p. 31).

Shuck. To cheat, lie, deceive.

Shuzzit. Marihuana.

1971: "I was blowing some good shuzzit." (Jones and Chilton, *Louis*, p. 114).

Sifter. Device for removing twigs and seeds from marihuana during cleaning.

Single. Marihuana cigarette.

1938: "Single." (Walton, *Marihuana*, p. 195).

Single Convention. United Nations agreement to limit, exclusively to medical and scientific purposes, the production, manufacture, export, import, distribution of, trade in, use and possession of certain drugs including the flowering or fruiting tops of the marihuana plant (excluding the seeds and leaves when not accompanied by the tops). The Single Convention was ratified by the United States in 1967. U.S. support of the Single Convention was urged strongly by antimarihuana forces such as H. J. Anslinger because relaxation of domestic laws against marihuana would then become an international embarrassment to the U.S.

Sinsemilla. Spanish word meaning without seeds; marihuana made from unpollinated female marihuana flowers. Potent. Sinsemilla is produced by separating male plants from females before latter can be fertilized.

1980: "My sinsemilla is selling for $40 an ounce." (Novak, *High Culture*, p. 103).

Sipping. Smoking marihuana.
1950: "A man was smoking a cigarette, only, he seemed to be sipping rather than inhaling its smoke." (Smith, *Anger*, p. 201).

Siva. Hindu god. Revered because he was said to have swallowed poison from the sea that otherwise would have destroyed mankind. Bhang (marihuana) is taken as part of a religious devotion to Siva since Hindus believe he is very fond of it. Siva is known as the Lord of Bhang because he is believed to have brought bhang from the Himalalayas for his devotees.

Sivaratri. Hindu festival commemorating marriage of god Siva. To celebrate, bhang (marihuana) is drunk.

Skin. Marihuana cigarette paper. *See* Bambu, Top, ZigZag.

Skinny. 1. Marihuana cigarette paper. 2. Thin marihuana cigarette.

Skoofer, Skoofus, Skrufer, Skrufus. Marihuana cigarette.
1972: "Skoofer." (Folb, *Black Argot*, p. 89).

Slap it around. *See* Spread the good news.

Slave Master. Water pipe for smoking marihuana.
1972: "Slave master." (Brennan, *Drugs*, p. 86).

Smoke. Marihuana.
1946: ". . . made crazy one night by a marijuana cigarette, by something called smoke or snow." (McCullers, *Ballad of Sad Café*, p. 788).
1962: " 'Are you drunk? . . . No. Not even on smoke.' " (Pritchie, *Savage Kick*, p. 36).
1971: "I have a lot of housewives, welfare broads, that's more smoke for me." (Woodley, *Dealer*, p. 12).
1976: "We got back into it in a small way, just to pay for our own smoke." (Sorfleet, "Dealing," p. 134).

Smash. Hash oil.*

Sneaky Peat. Marihuana mixed with wine.
1955: "Sneaky peat." (Braddy, "Narcotic Argot," p. 88).

Snop. Marihuana.

Soft drugs. Term used to distinguish drugs such as marihuana, which do not cause physical dependence, from those such as heroin, which do cause dependence.

1963: "Junk is pushed here—usually soft stuff: marihuana, pills—but you can also score for hard." (Rechy, *City of Night*, p. 24).

1969: ". . . marihuana is 'softer' and less perilous than the others." (*Time*, September 26, p. 68).

Sohl, Mrs. Ethel "Bunny." First (1938) to plead marihuana induced insanity as a defense in murder charge under newly passed Marihuana Tax Act (1937). The plea was not accepted. Sohl was sentenced to life imprisonment in New Jersey.

Sole. Flat, rectangular piece of hashish. So-called because hashish smugglers in North Africa used them as false soles in their shoes to avoid detection by customs guards.

Solid. Marihuana cigarette containing tobacco.

Soma. Mysterious drug mentioned in Hindu religious writings. Sometimes it has been interpreted as a reference to marihuana but usually as a reference to the mushroom, *Amanita muscaria.*

Son of One. Hash oil.* *See also* One.

1971: "The 'Son of One' was oil from Afghanistan." (*Marihuana Review*, vol. 1, no. 8, p. 23).

1977: ". . . 'Son of One,' seemed a bit less potent even though sellers claimed it was made from Afghani primo and quality Mexican weed." (*High Times*, February, p. 67).

Space Cadet. *See* Burned Out.

Spaced (out). Dazed from smoking marihuana; stuporous, disoriented.

1971: "This morning we got completely spaced before we even dressed." (Hall, *Heads*, p. 16).

Special. Potent marihuana cigarette.

1938: "Special." (Walton, *Marihuana*, p. 195).

1948: "Special: a slightly more potent and expensive marihuana cigarette." (Gottschalk and Cowdry, *Language*, p. 13).

Spiked. Tobacco cigarette to which marihuana has been added.

1937: "A man lit a 'spiked' cigarette." (Cooper, *Here's to Crime*, p. 335).

Spliff, Splim, Splint. Marihuana cigarette.

1967: "One could say I was at the beginning of a long and well-packed spliff." (Chaplin, *Grass*, p. 170).

1974: "There's nothing so gauche as having a well-made spliff dissolve at the seams." (Isyurhash and Rusoff, *Gourmet*, p. 52).

1977: "A man came up to me, and he gave me a spliff." (*High Times*, September, p. 48).

1979: "Four Rastas smoking spliffs will smoke four spliffs—one for each, no passing." (Nicholas, *Rastafari*, p. 49).

1980: ". . . one of the huge joints called a spliff." (Novak, *High Culture*, p. 211).

Split. To leave, depart.

Spread the good news, Slap it around. To offer a marihuana cigarette.

1954: "To offer doped cigarettes: to slap it about, to lay it on thickly or thinly, to spread the good news." (Bevan, *Everybody's*, June 12, p. 12).

Spring. To offer a marihuana cigarette.

Square. Conformist; nonuser of drugs.

1944: "If you ain't high, you feel square." (Marcovitz and Myers, "Marihuana Addict," p. 384).

Square Joint. Tobacco cigarette.

Squire's Extract. Preparation of marihuana made by English pharmacist Peter Squire. Squire and Sons became the primary and most reliable suppliers of marihuana extract in England in the late 1800s.

Squirrel. Store large amount of marihuana in a hiding place. *See* Stache.

Stache, Stash. Hidden supply of marihuana or any drug.

1955: "I stashed my stuff in someone's hall." (Braddy, "Anonymous Verses," p. 161).

1961: ". . . where he stashed his pot." (Hughes, *Fantastic Lodge*, p. 84).

1967: "The stash is the place where marihuana is kept or, more correctly, it is the hidden marihuana." (Rosevear, *Pot*, p. 62).

1968: "U.S. soldiers in Vietnam found a Viet Cong stash of marihuana worth about two hundred thousand dollars." (Gross, *Flower People*, p. 11).

1979: ". . . somebody else's special portable dope stash . . ." (Goldman, *Grass Roots*, p. 27).

Stack. Quantity of marihuana cigarettes.

1955: "Stack." (Braddy, "Narcotic Argot," p. 88).

Stash Container. Paraphernalia item. Container for storing marihuana.

Steam Roller. Empty toilet tissue roll used as steamboat.*
1970: "Steam roller." (Brennan, *Drugs*, p. 89).

Steamboat. Empty box, tube, or rolled paper, with a hole for marihuana cigarette. Its purpose is to keep smoke from dissipating so that
more can be inhaled.
1967: "This little contraption is called a steamboat because the roach
       looks like the smokestack in a steamboat." (*Newsweek*, July 24,
       p. 49).
1969: "The steamboat is a combination of a pipe and a joint merging
       the best of both into a powerful tool of good." (Margolis and
       Clorfene, *Grass*, p. 117).
1974: "A steamboat looks like a glass test tube with two holes punched
       in it." (Isyurhash and Rusoff, *Gourmet*, p. 58).

Stella. Brand of marihuana cigarette paper.

Stencil. Long, thin marihuana cigarette.
1972: "Stencil." (Folb, *Black Argot*, p. 89).

Stepped on. Marihuana adulterated with sugar or syrup to increase its
weight. *See* Sugared.
1974: "Stepped on." (Isyurhash and Rusoff, *Gourmet*, p. 34).

Stepping Stone Theory. Theory that marihuana leads to use of other
drugs.

Stick. Marihuana cigarette.
1938: "Some vipers get high on a single stick." (Berger, *New Yorker*,
       March 12, p. 48).
1944: "Good stuff will cost you $5 for two sticks." (Marcovitz and
       Myers, "Marihuana Addict," p. 383).
1951: "They are dried and made into cigarettes, commonly called
       reefers, muggles, or sticks." (*San Diego Evening Tribune*, July
       25, p. 17a).
1952: "Once a kid starts with a few sticks. . . ." (Oursler and Smith,
       Hooked, p. 32).
1953: "At seventy-five cents a stick, seventy sticks to the ounce, it
       sounded like money." (Burroughs, *Junkie*, p. 35).
1953: ". . . two sticks of pot." (Holmes, *Horn*, p. 56).
1955: ". . . his first stick of marihuana." (Ellson, *Reefer Boy*, p. 277).
1956: "You never really lit a stick?" (Hunter, *Second Ending*, p. 246).
1958: "He'd asked to roll a stick for me." (Kerouac, *Subterraneans*,
       p. 5).

1960: "They doped heavily, to the disgust of the older men, for whom whiskey, women, and an occasional stick of tea were all that a decent musician ever needed." (Newton, *Jazz Scene*, p. 221).

1960: "She took the stick down from her mouth." (De Mexico, *Marijuana Girl*, p. 46).

1967: "Red rolled two more sticks." (Chaplin, *Grass*, p. 133).

1968: ". . . stick of pot." (Thomas, *Mean Streets*, p. 65).

1970: "As soon as I lit up my first stick of hashish . . ." (Jamer, *Sex Communes*, p. 48).

Stinkweed. 1. Marihuana. 2. Jimsonweed.

Stoned. Under the influence of marihuana; very high*; immobile.

1956: "Man, he just dropped over—stoned." (Longstreet, *Real Jazz*, p. 146).

1958: ". . . when we're practically stoned . . ." (Kerouac, *Subterraneans*, p. 21).

1959: "He was stoned out of his mind with pot." (Lipton, *Holy Barbarians*, p. 85).

1961: "You never see anyone that's real stoned on pot." (Hughes, *Fantastic Lodge*, p. 73).

1967: "I closed the store, got stoned, and relaxed on my roof." (Ric, *Esquire*, September, p. 190).

1968: "It's not necessary for me to be stoned all the time." (Gross, *Flower People*, p. 9).

1971: "I stopped a coupla times to smoke a joint, so by the time I reached our house, I was pretty stoned." (Hall, *Heads*, p. 23).

Straight. 1. Non-drug user. *See* Square. 2. Not under the influence of drugs. 3. Under the influence of marihuana. 4. A tobacco cigarette.

1944: "His headaches were more frequent when he was 'straight.' " (Marcovitz and Myers, "Marihuana Addict," p. 384).

1946: "Does he get straight?" (Charen and Perelman, "Marihuana Addicts," p. 678).

1960: "Get straight." (De Mexico, *Marijuana Girl*, p. 153).

1960: "You save the roaches when they get too small to hold, wad them up, pick the tobacco from the end of a 'straight' (a regular cigarette), put in the wadded roach, crimp the end of the straight, and fire it up for one last drag." (Chiardi, *Saturday Review*, p. 12).

1961: "I had terrible eyes for a straight." (Hughes, *Fantastic Lodge*, p. 112).

1967: "With more and more middle class 'straights' joining the ranks of pot smokers . . ." (*Newsweek*, July 24, p. 49).

1969: "Heads and straights are both victims of their respective stereo-
    typing processes." (Spitzmiller, "Head Community," p. 2).
1972: "This is the first day I've been completely straight for a week."
    (Hall, *Heads*, p. 65).

Straighten out. Smoke marihuana.
1946: "How about straightening a guy out?" (Charen and Perelman,
    "Marihuana Addicts," p. 678).

Straw. Marihuana.

Street Dealer. Marihuana seller who deals in small quantities.

Stretch. To dilute a drug, for example, mix oregano with marihuana.

Stretch hemp. To be hanged.

Strung (out). 1. Dazed, disoriented, exhausted from drug use. 2. Using
drugs heavily.

Stuff. Marihuana or any drug.
1935: "The Stuff Is Here." Song recorded by Cleo Brown.

Sugared. Marihuana soaked in sugared water and then dried. Purpose
is to increase its apparent weight.
1967: "It was bad sugar-cured grass." (Ric, *Esquire*, September, p.
    101).

Sugar Weed. *See* Sugared.

Super Dope. Marihuana to which formaldehyde has been added.

Super Grass. Marihuana to which PCP (Phencyclidine) has been added.

Super Pot. Marihuana soaked in alcohol and then dried.

Supremo. Exceptionally high potency marihuana or hashish.

Sweet Lucy. Marihuana soaked or extracted in wine.
1948: "Sweet Lucy." (Gottschalk and Cowdry, *Language*, p. 14).

Sweet Lunch. Marihuana.
1967: "Sweet Lunch." (Siragusa, *Trail of the Poppy*, p. 235).

Sweet Mary. Marihuana.
1968: "More than half the men on one recent R & R flight to Australia
    were caught with Sweet Mary in their possession." (*Marihuana
    Review*, vol. 1, no. 1, p. 5).

Swinging. Uninhibited.

Swingle. To break hemp fibers.

Synethesia. Perception of sensations not normally associated with a stimulus, for example, hearing colors, seeing music.

Synhexyl. Synthetic marihuanalike compound developed and used in 1940s on an experimental basis to treat depression. Same as pyrahexyl.

Synthetic Marihuana. *See* THC.

T

T. *See* Tea.

T-Man. 1. Federal narcotics agent, short for treasury man. The treasury department was responsible for narcotics control until 1968, when narcotics control was placed under the justice department. 2. Marihuana smoker.
1936: "A 'T-man' is one who smokes marihuana." (Spencer, "Marihuana," p. 300).

Talk down. Reassure; calm; alleviate someone's drug-induced anxiety.

Tall. High,* stoned,* intoxicated on marihuana.

Taste. Smoke a sample marihuana cigarette before buying to determine potency and general quality.
1965: "The dealer opens each block and 'tastes' it, smoking a little to judge the quality." (*Village Voice*, December 1, p. 3).
1967: "After the buyer has examined the marihuana and rolled a cigarette, he will taste (smoke) it." (Rosevear, *Pot*, p. 31).
1971: "This usually meant going to the city in somebody's house, meeting a cat, tasting (trying) his stuff, and exchanging money for dope." (Hall, *Heads*, p. 19).

Taylor, Bayard (1825-1878). American writer and traveler. First American to describe the effects of hashish on himself. Two of his books, *A Journey to Central Africa* (1854) and *The Land of the Saracens, or, Pictures of Palestine, Asia Minor, Sicily and Spain* (1855) excited the imagination of American readers and influenced some of them, like Fitz Hugh Ludlow, to experiment with hashish.

Tea. Marihuana. From either the fact that shredded marihuana looked like loose tea leaves, or because marihuana was "sipped," or because tea was sometimes brewed with marihuana.
1930: "Tee Rollers Rub." Song recorded by Freddie Nicholson.
1931: "It is the cheapest and the weakest of all the preparations of hashish and is taken as 'tea.' " (Stanley, "Marihuana," p. 255).

1933: "Texas Tea Party." Music recorded by Benny Goodman.

1937: "We only work when we're high on tea." (Anslinger, "Marihuana," p. 150).

1940: "Three highballs and three sticks of tea." (Chandler, *Farewell,
My Lovely*, p. 60).

1945: "Perhaps it was due to all the 'tea' I smoked." (Marcovitz and
Myers, "Marihuana Addict," p. 391).

1952: "I'd rather stay with the Tea. It's great pod." (Mandell, *Flee the
Angry Strangers*, p. 135).

1953: ". . . lit up a stick of tea with the piano man." (Holmes, *Horn*,
p. 7).

1956: "A little tea every now and then—but never the big stuff."
(Marsten, *So Nude*, p. 86).

1958: ". . . sat on the floor in front of an open newspaper in which
the tea (poor quality L.A. but good enough) and rolled, or
twisted, . . ." (Kerouac, *Subterraneans*, p. 5).

1960: " 'Just a little tea,' he said." (King, *Enemy*, p. 24).

1961: "The average American citizen in an average community has
probably never heard of 'reefers' or 'tea' or other words in the
argot of marihuana users." (Anslinger and Oursler, *Murderers*,
p. 36).

Tea Bag. Marihuana cigarette.

Tea Blower. Marihuana user.

1952: "Tea blower." (Lannoy and Masterson, "Hophead Jargon," p.
30).

1970: "Tea blower." (Cromwell, *Slang*, p. 78).

Tea Head. Marihuana user.

1948: "Tea-head." (Gottschalk and Cowdry, *Language*, p. 14).

1953: "Tea heads are not junkies." (Burroughs, *Junkie*, p. 36).

Tea Hound. Marihuana user.

1942: "Tea hound." (Berrey and Bark, *Thesaurus*, p. 476).

1946: "They prefer the society of 'freaks' or 'tea hounds' to so-called
'squares.' " (Charren and Perelman, "Marihuana Addicts," p.
677).

1949: "Tea hound." (Monteleone, *Criminal Slang*, p. 234).

1951: "The subject of tea-hounds . . ." (Lait and Mortimer, *Washington Confidential*, p. 148).

Tea Pad. Place where marihuana is smoked.

1938: "Tea pad . . . place where reefer smokers congregate." (Yawger,
"Marihuana," p. 355).

1943: "The tea pad may be anything from a rented room to a suite in a fashionable hotel." (*Time*, July 19, p. 54).

1944: "A 'tea-pad' is a room or an apartment in which people gather to smoke marihuana. The majority of such places are located in the Harlem district. It is our impression that the landlord, the agent, the superintendent or the janitor is aware of the purposes for which the premises are rented.

The 'tea-pad' is furnished according to the clientele it expects to serve. Usually, each 'tea-pad' has comfortable furniture, a radio, victrola or, as in most instances, a rented nickelodeon. The lighting is more or less uniformly dim, with blue predominating. An incense burner is considered part of the furnishings. The walls are frequently decorated with pictures of nude subjects suggestive of perverted sexual practices. The furnishings, as described, are believed to be essential as a setting for those participating in smoking marihuana.

Most 'tea-pads' have their trade restricted to the sale of marihuana. Some places did sell marihuana and whiskey, and a few places also served as houses of prostitution." (*La Guardia Report*, pp. 9-10).

1957: "On another occasion I was in a 'tea pad' when it was actually raided by some holdup men." (Danforth and Horan, *Big City*, p. 128).

Tea Party. Gathering to smoke marihuana. Now called pot party.*

1945: "He used to go to 'tea parties' and 'viper pads' every other week." (Marcovitz and Myers, "Marihuana Addict," p. 384).

1946: "Everything went at a tea party." (Charen and Perelman, "Marihuana Addicts," p. 384).

Tea Shades. Dark glasses worn by marihuana smokers.

Tead up. Under the influence of marihuana.

1944: ". . . thinking about my 'boys' all tea-d up." (Marcovitz and Myers, "Marihuana Addict," p. 383).

Teeny-bopper. Ten- to fifteen-year-old girl.

1966: "The teeny-bopper on MacDougal Street who buys a 'nickle' (five dollars' worth) of marihuana and gets a nickle (five cents) of oregano has little recourse." (*Village Voice*, December 1, p. 21).

1968: ". . . it is the teenybopper's ready acceptance of drugs . . ." (*New York Times*, January 11, p. 18/7).

Temple Balls, Temple Bells, Temple Hash. Balls of hashish allegedly buried for seven years by Hindu holy men for later use in religious ceremonies. Now sold commercially.

1971: "... pressing it into temple bells with their palms ..." (Coyote Man, *Buzz*, p. 5).

1979: "Ten-ounce bags of Nepalese hashish are sometimes broken down into pellets before being formed into temple balls." (Cherniak, *Hashish*, p. 23).

1979: "It is moulded into sticks, fingers, disks, slaps and 'temple balls.' " (Goldman, *Grass Roots*, p. 54).

Teo. Marihuana smoker.

1949: "Teo." (Monteleone, *Criminal Slang*, p. 235).

Texas Leaguer. Marihuana smoker. *See* Texas Tea.

1959: "Texas leaguer." (Schmidt, *Narcotics*, p. 182).

Texas Tea. Marihuana.

1949: "Texas tea." (Monteleone, *Criminal Slang*, p. 235).

THC. Tetrahydrocannabinol. The principal psychoactive* ingredient in marihuana.

1969: "Something called THC appeared on the black market last summer." (*Time*, January 24, p. 58).

Thai Sticks. Marihuana originating from Thailand. So-called because it is formed from tops of marihuana plants wound around sticks of bamboo which are then bound together. Very potent and expensive.

1975: "Thai sticks are enjoying unprecedented popularity." (*High Times*, October, p. 43).

1978: "Thai sticks are essentially a marketing gimmick." (*Playboy*, September, p. 220).

1979: "Thai sticks, the most popular grass in New York ..." (Goldman, *Grass Roots*, p. 27).

1980: "Connoisseurs complain that 'Thai stick' has become a meaningless phrase ..." (Novak, *High Culture*, p. 191).

Thai Weed. Marihuana from Thailand.

There. High,* intoxicated on marihuana.

Thing. Marihuana cigarette.

1967: "The most popular method of marihuana smoking is handmade cigarettes called ... things." (Rosevear, *Pot*, p. 64).

Thirteen. Marihuana cigarette.

Thriller. Marihuana cigarette.
1938: ". . . when you smoke a thriller." (St. Johns, "Walking," p. 105).

Throw me out with. Give me a marihuana cigarette.
1972: "Throw me out with." (Folb, *Black Argot*, p. 146).

Thumb. Fat marihuana cigarette. *See also* Bomber.
1969: "Big fat joints are called Bombers or Thumbs." (Margolis and Clorfene, *Grass*, p. 103).

Thunder Weed. Marihuana.
1935: "Thunder weed." (Pollock, *Underworld Speaks*, p. 30).

Tich. *See* THC.
1974: "Everyone in my town is snorting what they say is THC . . . or 'Tich.' " (*High Times*, vol. 1, no. 2, p. 8).

Tighten your wig. Smoke marihuana (1930s). *See* Wig.

Tin. Container of marihuana. *See* Can.
1937: "You could buy a whole tobacco tin of the stuff for 50 cents." (Anon., "Marihuana," p. 186).
1937: ". . . he poured from a tobacco tin—elongated cans used for a cheap brand of smoking tobacco are almost the inevitable container for marihuana in bulk." (Cooper, *Here's to Crime*, p. 335).

Tin Action. Purchase of tin of marihuana. *See also* Can Action.

Tincture. Most commonly used marihuana preparation in medicines prior to 1920s.

Toak, Toat. *See* Toke.

Toke. To inhale marihuana smoke.
1952: "Toke." (Lannoy and Masterson, "Hophead Jargon," p. 30).
1968: "She takes another toke and gazes proprietorially around the room." (Gross, *Flower People*, p. 22).
1970: "After three or four hundred tokes, the Yippies knew they were high." (Sanders, *Shards*, p. 27).
1971: "After one or two tokes I felt a wave of relief through my body." (Hall, *Heads*, p. 27).
1971: "Empty your lungs completely, then slowly but steadily toke." (*Marihuana Review*, vol. 1, no. 6, p. 1).
1979: "No grass in the world can still get you off in three tokes." (Goldman, *Grass Roots*, p. 112).

1980: ". . . two tokes of dynamite weed . . ." (Novak, *High Culture*, p. 186).

Toke Pipe. Short-stemmed pipe for smoking marihuana.

Toke up. To light a marihuana cigarette.

Toker. 1. Marihuana smoker. 2. Glass pipe for smoking marihuana.

Tolerance. Adaptation of the body to the point where more of a given drug is required to produce the same intensity of experience as that felt when first using it.

Top. Brand of marihuana cigarette paper—pot spelled backwards.

Torch. Marihuana cigarette.
1977: "Torch." (Lentini, *Vice*, p. 144).

Torch up. To light a marihuana cigarette.
1955: "Torch up." (Braddy, "Narcotic Argot," p. 88).

Torpedo. Thick marihuana cigarette. *See also* Bomber, Thumb.
1943: ". . . the cigarets (sic) were neatly rolled, up to full strength, free of seed and stems, and sized in accord with the customers' specifications from long 'torpedos' to little twisted reefers." (*Life*, July 19, p. 83/2).

Tote. *See* Toke.

Tow. Coarse fibers left over after hemp fibers have been removed from stalks.

Trafficking. Selling marihuana or any other drug.

Treat a J. Add other drugs to a marihuana cigarette. *See also* A(tom) Bomb, Candy a J.

Trichome. Structure on marihuana leaf that produces THC-containing resin.

Trigger. To smoke marihuana after taking LSD.

Trip. Feelings resulting from use of marihuana or psychedelic drugs.
1968: "You can trip on marihuana." (Gross, *Flower People*, p. 3).
1970: "Many of the soldiers who were smoking pot heavily likened these 'trips' to those produced by LSD." (Kaplan, "Marihuana," p. 262).
1970: ". . . a distilled essence of hashish that was the most potent trip anyone had ever witnessed." (Sanders, *Shards*, p. 11).

Trip Grass. Marihuana to which amphetamine has been added.

T-Timers. Dark glasses worn by marihuana smokers.
1952: "T-timers." (Lannoy and Masterson, "Hophead Jargon," p. 3).

Tube. Marihuana cigarette.
1937: "Then, lighting the tube, he took a few puffs." (Cooper, *Here's to Crime*, p. 335).

Tuck and roll. Fold ends of marihuana cigarette instead of twisting them.

Tuned in. Aware; involved; knowledgeable.

Turkey. To inhale marihuana smoke through the nose.
1970: "Turkey." (Gardner, "Slang," p. 26).
1971: "To turkey it, you clamp the roach between the heads of two paper matches." (U. California, *Folklore*, p. 162).

Turn on. 1. Initiate someone into marihuana use. 2. To use marihuana.
1953: "We kept the weed in Mary's apartment, turned her on for all she could use, and gave her a 50 percent commission on sales." (Burroughs, *Junkie*, p. 36).
1956: "Some more guys turned me on when I was just a kid." (Duke, *Sideman*, p. 274).
1960: "Going to turn on man?" (De Mexico, *Marijuana Girl*, p. 45).
1961: "One night some cats turned us on for the first time." (Hughes, *Fantastic Lodge*, p. 71).
1963: "I remember a party where the three of us turned on with marihuana." (Rechy, *City of Night*, p. 406).
1964: "I turned on when I was fourteen." (Harris, *Junkie Priest*, p. 2).
1965: "If everyone at the party 'turns on' the atmosphere is subdued." (*New York Post*, December 3, p. 45).
1967: "I had my first turn-on in the first few hours of 1964." (Chaplin, *Grass*, p. 170).

Turn on, tune in, drop out. Slogan of hippie "flower children" of the 1960s, meaning take drugs, become aware, renounce the materialistic world.

Turned on. High,* under the influence of marihuana.

Twig. Marihuana.
1970: "Twig." (Cromwell, *Slang*, p. 76).

Twist. Marihuana cigarette. From the twisted ends of marihuana cigarette, needed to keep the loose material from falling out.

1936: "Twist." (Maurer, "Argot of Underworld," p. 127).
1951: "So far as students are concerned, teachers might well be suspicious if they begin to catch words like 'reefer,' 'twist,' 'weed,' and 'tea' for most addicts start with marihuana." (*National Education Association Journal*, May, p. 342/2).

Twist a dream. To roll a marihuana cigarette.
1949: "Twist a dream." (Monteleone, *Criminal Slang*, p. 245).

Twist a giraffe's tail. To smoke marihuana.
1959: "Twist a giraffe's tail." (Schmidt, *Narcotics*, p. 185).

Twister. Marihuana user.
1936: "Twister: One who rolls his own twists, or marihuana cigarettes." (Maurer, "Argot of Underworld," p. 127).
1946: "Those who roll their own cigarettes for economy are twisters." (Maurer, Narcotic Addict," p. 572).
1949: "Twister." (Monteleone, *Criminal Slang*, p. 245).

U

Uncle. Federal narcotics officer.

Up. High,* intoxicated, exhilarated.
1946: "How long since you been up there?" (Charen and Perelman, "Marihuana Addicts," p. 678).

Uptight. Nervous, anxious, tense.

User. Marihuana user.

V

Van Linschoten, John Huyghen. Sixteenth-century Dutch traveler and writer. His book, *Itinerario*, published in 1596, was a best-seller of its day. It was one of the first popular books to describe the effects of cannabis, although much of his description of the effects of the drug was plagiarized from an earlier book by Garcia daOrta.* Van Linschoten also deliberately exaggerated the effects of the drug, and, as a result of his book, many people got the mistaken impression that cannabis and opium had identical effects.

Van Rheede, H. Dutch author (*Hortus Malabaricus*, 1678). First writer to publish a drawing of the marihuana plant.

Vegged out. *See* Burned Out.

Vibes. Vibrations; feelings concerning someone or something.

Vipe. To smoke marihuana.
1936: ". . . to 'vipe' is to smoke marijuana." (Spencer, "Marihuana," p. 300).
1946: "It takes time and practice to vipe satisfactorily." (Maurer, "Narcotic Addict," p. 573).

Viper. Marihuana user. Term self-imposed by marihuana users in 1930s. Possibly originating from term "snake (viper) in the grass."
1935: "Viper's Moan." Song recorded by Willie Bryant.
1938: "If You're a Viper." Song recorded by Bob Howard.
1938: "Vipers sometimes carry a little bag of peppermint or peanuts." (Berger, *New Yorker*, March 12, p. 48).
1943: "Etiquette between pushers and vipers is necessarily delicate." (*Time*, July 19, p. 54).
1952: "What kind of viper are you, drinking beer and whiskey all the time?" (Mandell, *Flee the Angry Strangers*, p. 340).
1955: *"Since ma was a Viper*
And daddy would snort
There wasn't much more
I had to be taught."
(Braddy, "Anonymous Verses," p. 134).

Viper Song. Song about marihuana, for example, "Song of the Vipers," "Smokin' Reefers," "Chant of the Weed."

Viper's Weed. Marihuana.

Viperish. Fond of marihuana.
1953: "He scores for a few good 'cats' and 'chicks' because he is viperish." (Burroughs, *Junkie*, p. 31).

Vonce. Marihuana butt. *See also* Roach.
1965: "The butt of the cigarette, or 'vonce' is saved and used in emergencies when fresh marihuana is not available." (Winick, "Marihuana," p. 233).

W

Wacky Tobaccy. Marihuana.

Wacky Weed, Whacky Weed. Potent marihuana from Colombia; black in color.

1974: "Colombian wacky weed." (*High Times*, vol. 1, no. 2, p. 39).

1980: "The most famous of the dark Colombians is wacky weed, a legendary variety said to make everything absurd." (Novak, *High Culture*, p. 190).

Wahegan. Potent marihuana from Hawaii.

Waste. 1. To smoke completely. 2. To kill.

1967: "I decided to go upstairs to my place and waste a stick of pot." (Thomas, *Mean Streets*, p. 220).

Wasted. Very intoxicated on marihuana, to the point of lethargy.

1970: "Wasted." (Goode, *Marihuana Smokers*, p. 329).

Water Pipe. Pipe in which smoke is drawn through water to cool it and remove impurities.

Way down. Needing marihuana (1930s-1940s).

Weed. Marihuana.

1928: "Emit sour notes after smoking weed." (*Chicago Tribune*, July 1, p. 12/3).

1931: "Chant of the Weeds." Song recorded by Don Redman.

1934: "Have a weed, English?" (De Lenoir, *Hundredth Man*, p. 226).

1937: "It now is being called . . . 'weed.' " (Cooper, *Here's to Crime*, p. 333).

1940: " 'Red' Caldwell bought two 'weeds.' " (Himes, *Esquire*, March, p. 58).

1945: "I can do without coffee, I can do without tea, but I sure can't do without my weed." (Saxon, *Gumbo*, p. 462).

1953: "Herman told me about a kilo of first class New Orleans' weed." (Burroughs, *Junkie*, p. 30).

1955: "I don't smoke weed." (Ellson, *Rock*, p. 47).

1958: "Blasting weed was fine." (Braddy, "Anonymous Verses," p. 130).

1977: "About the second time I smoked weed I got higher than a kite." (Rettig, *Manny*, pp. 32-33).

Weed Eater. Marihuana user. *See also* Weed Head, Weed Hound, Weed Twister.

Weed Head. Marihuana user. *See also* Weed Hound, Weed Twister.
1933: "His brother, who is a reported 'weed head' . . ." (Hayes and
      Bowery, "Marihuana," p. 1095).
1949: "Weed head." (Monteleone, *Criminal Slang*, p. 250).
1951: "All weed-heads are cop haters." (Lait and Mortimer, *Washing-
      ton Confidential*, p. 147).
1966: "Adolescent 'weed heads' (regular marihuana users) maintain-
      ing the appearance of 'being cool'. . ." (Sutter, "Righteous Dope
      Fiend," p. 179).

Weed Hound. Marihuana user.
1949: "Weed hound." (Monteleone, *Criminal Slang*, p. 250).

Weed Twister. 1. Marihuana user. 2. Person who borrows small amounts of marihuana.
1935: "Weed twister." (Pollock, *Underworld Speaks*, p. 30).

Weedly. Female marihuana smoker.
1955: "Weedly." (Braddy, "Narcotic Argot," p. 88).

Weekend Doper, Habit, Tripper, User. Casual marihuana or drug user.
1969: "The head is not to be confused with the recreational user,
      the weekend tripper who enjoys an occasional furtive joint and
      returns to a conventional white-collar job on Monday morning."
      (Spitzmiller, "Head Community," p. 1).
1974: "To the beginner, or 'weekend doper,' the most rewarding
      effects happen on the sensual level." (Isyurhash and Rusoff,
      Gourmet, p. 80).

Whacky Tobacky. *See* Wacky Tobaccy.

Wheat. Marihuana.

Wheaties. Marihuana cigarette paper.

Where's Mary? Where can I get marihuana?
1952: "Where's Mary?" (Lannoy and Masterson, "Hophead Jargon,"
      p. 30).

Whiskers. Police.

Whittier, John Greenleaf. American poet. First American to write about hashish. His poem "The Haschish," part of his *Anti-Slavery*

Poems (1854), describes the hallucinations and muddled thinking associated with hashish use.

"Of all that Orient lands can vaunt
Of marvels with our own competing
The strangest is the Haschish plant
And what will follow on its eating."

Wig. Mind.
1961: "Everybody turned on and got stoned out of their wigs." (Hughes, *Fantastic Lodge*, p. 145).

Wigged (out). Loss of self-control.
1961: "When you really feel wigged." (Hughes, *Fantastic Lodge*, p. 74).
1965: "These guys who wig out . . ." (*New York Post*, December 3, p. 45).

Wild Weed. Marihuana growing wild; generally of low potency.
1976: "Picking wildweed can be dangerous sheriff-wise." (*High Times*, March, p. 8).

Wiped out. Very intoxicated.
1972: "Wiped out." (Smith and Gray, *It's So Good*, p. 208).

Wired. High* on marihuana.
1974: "When smoked, good shit will wire one up for thirty minutes to five hours." (Isyurhash and Rusoff, *Gourmet*, p. 17).

Woodward, Dr. William C. Physician and lawyer. A representative of the American Medical Association at the Taxation on Marihuana Hearings in 1937. Woodward was the only witness to speak out against imposition of a taxation bill that effectively outlawed marihuana. *See also* Marijuana Tax Act.

Wooten Report. British commission headed by Baroness Wooten to study the effects of marihuana. The committee concluded that marihuana was a relatively benign drug and recommended decriminalization and recognition that marihuana had legitimate medical uses (1968).

Wrecked. *See* Wasted.
1971: "He's only nice to me when he's wrecked." (Hall, *Heads*, p. 13).
1980: "We were both wrecked." (Novak, *High Culture*, p. 30).

Y

Yerba. Marihuana. From Spanish *herba*, meaning "weed."
1967: "I've been blasting yerba." (Thomas, *Mean Streets*, p. 112).

Yesca. Marihuana.
1952: "Yesca." (Lannoy and Masterson, "Hophead Jargon," p. 31).
1955: "Yesca." (Braddy, "Narcotic Argot," p. 88).
1977: "Yesca." (Lentini, *Vice*, p. 145).

Youngblood. Beginning marihuana smoker.

Z

Zacatecas Purple. Potent marihuana from Mexico.

Zig Zag. Brand of marihuana cigarette paper.
1969: "The first time you buy Zig Zag is very much like the first time you bought a little tin of three condoms." (Margolis and Clorfene, *Grass*, p. 100).
1969: "I stopped at the grass counter and asked for some regular white zig-zag cigarette rolling papers." (*Time*, September 26, p. 73).

Zig Zag Man. Man depicted on Zig Zag paper.

Zol. Marihuana cigarette. Term primarily used in South Africa; *see* appendix.
1955: "Zol." (Braddy, "Narcotic Argot," p. 88).

Zonked. Under the influence of marihuana; very high.*
1967: "One night when I was completely zonked out on hash." (*Marihuana Review*, vol. 1, no. 1, p. 3).
1968: "I was so zonked . . ." (Gross, *Flower People*, p. 45).
1968: "I was really zonked the other night." (U. California, *Folklore*, p. 18).
1979: ". . . zonked and deliriously happy . . ." (Goldman, *Grass Roots*, p. 116).

Zooie. Cylindrical device for holding butt of marihuana cigarette.

Zoom. Marihuana to which PCP has been added.

Z-kit. Paraphernalia item consisting of marihuana pipe, roach clip, book of matches, and various other accessories.

APPENDIX: FOREIGN WORDS AND EXPRESSIONS ABOUT MARIHUANA

A

Aap. Marihuana (South Africa).
Aburi. Marihuana (Nigeria).
Afrogras. Marihuana (Nigeria).
Alcanque. Hemp (Portugal).
Algo. Marihuana (Costa Rica), literally "something."
Al-quinnab. Hashish (Arabic), literally "daughter of cannabis."
Amarilla, La. Marihuana (Colombia, Costa Rica), literally "the yellow one."
Anada. Marihuana (India), literally "joy."
Anasha. Marihuana (Russia).
Aparato. Marihuana (Costa Rica), literally "apparatus."
Asa. Hemp (Japan).
Asarath. Hashish (Turkey).
Assis. Hashish (Egypt, sixteenth century).
Assyouni. *See* Chatsraky.
Atchie Erva. Marihuana (Brazil).
Azallua. Hemp (Assyria, seventh century B.C.).

B

Bang. Marihuana (Persia, Brazil). *See* Bhang.
Banga. Marihuana (Iran). *See* Bhang.

Bangi. Marihuana (Iran). *See* Bhang.

Bangue. Marihuana (Hindu). *See* Bhang.

Banj. General term for narcotics (Arabic).

Bareta. Marihuana (Cuba).

Basiado. Marihuana (Brazil).

Bautizado. Marihuana adulterated with other substances (Costa Rica), literally "baptized."

Bendj. Marihuana (Coptic). *See* Bhang.

Beng. Marihuana (Persia). *See* Bhang.

Benghie. Marihuana (Egypt). *See* Bhang.

Benj. Marihuana (Arabic). *See* Bhang.

Berch. Hashish confection made with hashish, honey, and water (Egypt).

Bers. Electuary of hashish, opium, and syrup (Egypt).

Bhang. Marihuana (India). Origin of cognates Bang, Bendj, Benj, etc. Refers either to dried broken leaves, small stalks, and some flowers of marihuana plant, or, more often, to a beverage made with marihuana leaves, the most popular way of consuming the drug in India. Plants from which bhang is made receive relatively little attention during the growing season in contrast to plants used to make charas* and ganga.*

Bhanga. Marihuana (early Sanskrit, India). *See* Bhang.

Bicho. Marihuana (Costa Rica), literally "insect."

Bird's Tongue. Black gelatinous candy confection containing hashish, sugar, and spices (Egypt).

Birra. Marihuana (Brazil).

Bonita, La. Marihuana (Costa Rica), literally "pretty one."

C

Cachimba de Don Juan, La. Pipe for smoking marihuana (Costa Rica), literally "the pipe of Don Juan."

Canab. Hemp (Brittany).

Canaib. Hemp (Ireland).

Canamazo. Hemp (Mexico).

Canamo. Hemp (Spain).

Canapa. Hemp (Italy).

Canapis. Hemp (Rumania).

Canappa. Hemp (Spain).

Canapu. Hemp (Italy).

Canep. Hemp (Albania).

Cangonha. Marihuana (Brazil).

Canhamo. Hemp (Portugal).

Cerrado. Intoxicated by marihuana (Costa Rica), literally "uncomprehending."

Chanvre. Hemp (France).

Charas. Hashish (India). Consists of resin from marihuana plant.

Plants are carefully cultivated in rows, and the earth is periodically fertilized and tilled. During growing season, the plants are thinned to allow bushy growth. Male plants are pulled out as soon as their sex can be distinguished.

Up until the nineteenth century, in Nepal, naked workers walked through marihuana fields, periodically stopping to scrape resin from their bodies with a blunt instrument which would then be placed into a container. In India, much the same gathering process occurred except that the workers wore leather aprons instead of being nude.

In the current method of collection, workers pass through fields of ripe marihuana plants and fondle each flower. The resin gathers on their hands, and this is rolled into a wad and deposited into a container worn around the neck. The containers are brought to another worker who removes the contents, separates out any twigs or seeds, mixes it with a small amount of butter, and kneads it in a stone trough into a dense paste.

Chastry. *See* Chatsraky.

Chatsraky, Chatzraki. Mixture of hashish and wine to which henbane, nutmeg, essense of rose, vanilla, cantharides, and nux vomica are added (Egypt). Also called chastry and assyouni.

Cheio. Marihuana (Brazil).

Chicharra. Marihuana and tobacco cigarette (Cuba).

Chingas. Marihuana cigarette butt, "roach" (Costa Rica), literally "small amount."

Chira. Hemp (Greece).

Chochando. Intoxicated with marihuana, "high" (Costa Rica), literally "senile."

Chu Tsao, Chu Tso. Hemp (China).

Cochinada, La. Marihuana (Costa Rica), literally "filth."

Colilla. Marihuana cigarette butt, "roach" (Costa Rica), literally "butt." *See* Chingas.

Con las pilas puestas. Intoxicated with marihuana, "high" (Costa Rica), literally "with the batteries charged." *See also* Chochando.

Cosa, La. Marihuana (Costa Rica), literally "thing."

Crocodile's Penis. Hashish confection which at one time contained crocodile penis to enhance alleged aphrodisiac effects of hashish (Egypt).

 D

Dagga, Dakka. Marihuana (South Africa).

Dagga Rooker. Marihuana smoker (South Africa).

Dai ando. Marihuana (Vietnam).

Dawamesc. Hashish confection containing hashish, butter, cantharides, pistachio, musk, sugar, cinnamon, ginger, and cloves. Hashish is simmered in butter, mixture is strained, and ingredients are added to the extract (Arab countries). The famous "green paste" eaten by members of the Club des Haschischins.

Daxab. Marihuana (South Africa).

Desmoto. No longer under the influence of marihuaná (Costa Rica), literally "clear away."

Diamba. Marihuana (West Africa, Brazil).

Diambista. Marihuana (Brazil).

Dimbo. Marihuana (Gabon).

Doctor. Marihuana dealer (Costa Rica). *See also* El que receta, Medico, Pacientes.

Dok. Marihuana (Laos).

Don Juan, Dona Juanita. Marihuana (Mexico, Brazil).

Dumo. Marihuana (Gabon).

E

El que receta. Marihuana dealer (Costa Rica), literally "He who prescribes." *See also* Doctor, Medico.

Elva. Marihuana (Brazil).

En juanado. Under the influence of marihuana (Mexico).

En Lenado. Under the influence of marihuana (Central America), literally "in wool."

En Motado. Under the influence of marihuana (Central America).

En Yedado. Under the influence of marihuana (Central America).

Engaletado. Hidden supply of marihuana, "stash" (Costa Rica).

Erimo Seleke. Marihuana (Nigeria).

Erva. Marihuana (Brazil).

Esar. Mixture of hashish, tobacco, syrup, sugar, and honey (Turkey).

Esta Carajoda. Marihuana (Costa Rica), literally "damned thing."

Estar muy cerrado. Very intoxicated with marihuana, "stoned" (Costa Rica), literally "very uncomprehending."

Ewe Ajiwere. Marihuana (Nigeria).

Ewe Eva. Marihuana (Nigeria).

F

Femea. Marihuana (Brazil).

Fogonata. Smoking several marihuana cigarettes consecutively (Costa Rica), literally "bonfire."

Fumo Bravo. Marihuana (Brazil), literally "brave smoke."

Fumo de Angola. Marihuana (Brazil), literally "smoke of Angola."

Fumo de Caboclo. Marihuana (Brazil).

G

Gai Ando. Marihuana (Vietnam).

Gancho. Dishonest marihuana seller (Costa Rica), literally "hook."

Gandia. Marihuana (Mauritius).

Gandshakini. Marihuana confection consisting of marihuana, opium, and camphor (India).

Ganga. Hashish (Hindu).

Gangica. Hashish (India, Sanskrit).

Ganja. Hashish (India, Jamaica, Costa Rica). Dried flowering tops of female marihuana plant. Like charas,* the plants are carefully cultivated. The earth is tilled and manured. The plants are thinned to allow for bush growth. Male plants are uprooted as soon as their sex is evident. The plants are harvested when flowers are about finished producing resin. At that time, the plants are cut close to earth and laid on ground for a few hours. Flowers are removed before or after the plant is cut. Two types of ganja are made in India—round and flat.

Round ganja consists of flowers of the best-formed plants. The tops are kneaded in the palms of the hand into a resinous mass, which is formed into a cone and then left to dry.

Flat ganja consists of flowers that are removed and allowed to dry overnight. Dried flowers are then gathered into a pressing area and bare-footed workers trample over them, forming a gooey mass that is periodically removed and formed into flat slabs.

Ganzar. Hashish and opium mixture (Persia).

Garawisch. Similar to dawamesc.* Electuary of leaves and flowers of marihuana plant to which pistachio, musk, sugar, nutmeg, cardamom, and almonds are added (Arab countries).

Gard. Hashish powder (India).

Gashgish. Hashish (Persia).

Gem. Marihuana (Nigeria).

Gingi. Marihuana (Malabar).

Ginjeh. Marihuana (Java).

Ginji. Marihuana (Bengal).

Gongo. Marihuana (Brazil).

Goni. Marihuana (Sanskrit, India).

Goza. Water pipe for smoking hashish (Arab countries).

Grifa. Marihuana (Mexico, Costa Rica).

Guaza. Marihuana (India).

Guinnjeh. Marihuana (Java).

Gungeon. Marihuana (Jamaica).

Gunja. Hashish (Sanskrit).

Gunsche. Marihuana (Jamaica, Java).

Gurdu: Hashish (Kashmir).

H

Hachaichi. Hashish (Algeria).

Haenep. Hemp (Old English).

Hafioun. Hashish (Turkey).

Hampa. Hemp (Denmark, Sweden).

Hampr. Hemp (Finland).

Hanf. Hemp (Germany).

Hanpr. Hemp (Norway).

Hashache. Hashish (Egypt).
Hashish. Hashish (Arab countries). Resin from marihuana plant containing some flower parts but very little leaves. May contain oil to bind it together. Usually rolled into lumps or balls. Also called Hachisch, Hadschisch, Haschich, Haschisch, Hatchisch, and Haschischa.
Hembra, La. Female marihuana plant (Mexico), literally "female."
Hen-nab. Hemp (Arabic).
Hennep. Hemp (Holland).
Hennup. Hemp (Holland).
Herbe. Marihuana (France).
Hierba. Marihuana (Costa Rica, Cuba, Mexico), literally "grass," "weed."
Hoja. Marihuana (Colombia), literally "leaf."

I

Ibat al quinbus. Hashish (Arabic), literally "daughter of cannabis."
Ibn al quinnab. Hashish (Arabic), literally "son of cannabis."
Igbo. Marihuana (Nigeria).
Indian Tyre. Marihuana (Nigeria).
Indracana. Marihuana (India), literally "India's food."
Indrasans. Marihuana (India).
Injaga. Marihuana (Rwanda).
Insangu, Instasangu. Marihuana (Southwest Africa).

J

Jaya. Marihuana (India), literally "victorious."
Jia. Marihuana (India).
Josah. Pipe for smoking marihuana (Egypt).
Juana. Marihuana (Mexico).
Juanita. Marihuana (Mexico).

K

Kabak. Hashish (Turkey).
Kaif. Hashish (Russia).
Kaifirovat. Intoxicated with marihuana (Russia).
Kajola. Marihuana (Nigeria).
Kajolowo. Marihuana (Nigeria).
Kali. Marihuana (Hindu, Jamaica).
Kamp. Hemp (Denmark).
Kampe. Marihuana (Nigeria).
Kanabira. Hemp (Syria).
Kanapis. Hemp (Lithuania).
Kanaq. Hemp (Armenia).
Kancha. Hemp (Thailand).

Kaneder. Hemp (Arabic).
Kanep. Hemp (Albania).
Kang Cha. Marihuana (Thailand).
Kannab. Hemp (Persia).
Kannapis. Hemp (Greece).
Kanop. Hemp (Armenia).
Kanopj. Hemp (Poland).
Kanub. Hemp (Arabic).
Keij. Hashish (Kashmir).
Kemp. Hemp (Belgium).
Kender. Hemp (Hungary, Turkey).
Kenevir. Hemp (Bulgaria).
Kennevir. Hemp (Turkey).
Khan Cha. Marihuana (Cambodia).
Kief. Hashish (Morocco, North Africa).
Kif. Hashish (Morocco, North Africa).
Kinab. Hemp (Arabic).
Kinnabi. Hemp (Arabic).
Kinnabis. Hemp (Malaya).
Kinnub. Hemp (Ceylon).
Konneb. Hemp (Arabic).
Konop. Hemp (Bulgaria).
Konopie. Hemp (Poland).
Konopj. Hemp (Poland).
Konople. Hemp (Russia).
Konoplja. Hemp (Russia).
Kukuge. Marihuana (Nigeria).
Kunubu. Hemp (Assyria).
Kwane. Hemp (Central America).

L

Lebake. Marihuana (Central Africa).
Leno. Marihuana (Central America).
Liamba. Marihuana (Brazil).
Lily. Marihuana (Nigeria).
Los de la onda. Marihuana smokers (Costa Rica), literally "those of the wave," "tuned in."
Lutki. Marihuana concoction made of bhang* and alcohol (India).

M

Ma. Marihuana (China).
Ma'agoun. Hashish concoction made with 10% hashish melted in oil and mixed

with sugar, honey, butter, chocolate, and spices. Mixture is kneaded with powdered gum arabic and rolled into pills which are chewed (Egypt).

Ma'goungy. Person who prepares hashish confections (Egypt).

Ma jen. Marihuana seeds (China).

Ma pen. Marihuana pods (China).

Ma po. Marihuana flowers (China).

Macho. Male marihuana plant (Mexico).

Maconha. Marihuana (Brazil).

Macumba. Marihuana (Brazil).

Madjun. Hashish confection made by extracting hashish in simmering butter and adding spices to extract (North Africa). *See also* Ma'agoun.

Madjoun. Hashish confection containing hashish, tobacco, and syrup (Algeria, Turkey). *See also* Ma'agoun.

Majoan. Hashish confection containing hashish, opium, and datura (India). *See also* Ma'agoun.

Majoom, Majoon. Marihuana confection made by sautéing bhang* in butter. Resins rise to top of butter, forming a jelly that is cooled and removed and mixed with sugar, milk, honey, henbane, datura, and flavorings and heated. Mixture is cooled again, formed into a paste, and cut into small pieces which are chewed (India). *See also* Ma'agoun.

Maju. Marihuana beverage containing marihuana, opium, datura, mandrake, sugar, and spices (India, Turkey).

Malach. Hashish (Turkey).

Malban. Hashish confection containing hashish, sugar, and gelatin made into square pieces. Also called Turkish Delight (Egypt).

Malva. Marihuana (Brazil).

Manzoul. *See* Ma'agoun.

Mapouchari, Mapuchari. Hashish confection made with hashish, butter, and aromatic substances (Egypt).

Maria Johanna. Marihuana (Mexico).

Maricas. Pipe for smoking marihuana (Brazil).

Marilu. Marihuana (Costa Rica).

Mariquita. Marihuana (Costa Rica).

Maschechel. Cafe for smoking hashish (Egypt, Turkey).

Mashada. Marihuana (Mombasa).

Maslac. Hashish (Turkey).

Masmoch. *See* Ma'agoun.

Mata. Marihuana (Central Africa, Costa Rica).

Matokwane. Marihuana (Central Africa).

Mbange, Mbanze. Marihuana (Southern Africa).

Medico. Marihuana seller (Costa Rica), literally "doctor."

Momea. Marihuana (Tibet).

Mona. Female marihuana plant (Colombia).

Mora. Marihuana (Mexico).

Morisquita. Marihuana (Mexico).

Morocco. Marihuana (Nigeria).

Morrao. Marihuana (Brazil).
Moscorrofia. Marihuana (Costa Rica).
Mota. Marihuana (Mexico).
Moz. Hashish confection containing hashish and sugar (Egypt).
Muta. Marihuana (Mexico).

N

Narghile. Water pipe for smoking hashish (Iran, Turkey).
Nena. Marihuana (Mexico).
Njemu. Marihuana (East Africa, Tanganyika).
Nsangu. Marihuana (Zulu).

O

Oja. Marihuana (Nigeria).
Omo ile. Marihuana (Nigeria).

P

Pacientes. Marihuana user (Costa Rica), literally "patient." *See also* Doctor, Medico.
Pajuela. Marihuana (Mexico).
Pango. Marihuana (Brazil).
Pantoufle. Sole-shaped cake of hashish, weighing a quarter of a kilogram. The shape was due to smugglers cutting and pressing hashish to fit into shoes and inserting them beneath the sole of the foot so as to escape detection. After the trick was detected, the practice ceased, but the shape was retained as indicative of superior hashish (Egypt).
Papirosa. Cigarette made with hashish (Russia).
Penka. Hemp (Russia).
Phulganja. Marihuana (Southern Africa).
Pitillo. Marihuana cigarette (Costa Rica).
Planta da felicidade. Marihuana (Brazil), literally "plant of happiness."
Poddar. "Ganja doctor." Individual who removes male marihuana plants as soon as they are detectable (India). *See* Ganja.
Potacion de guaya. Marihuana soaked in wine or brandy (Mexico), literally "drink of grief."
Potaguaya. Marihuana (Portugal).
Putti. Marihuana (India).

Q

Quemadero. Gathering place to smoke marihuana (Costa Rica), literally "burning place."

Quemadores. Marihuana smokers (Costa Rica), literally "burners."
Quemarla. Smoke marihuana (Costa Rica), literally "burn it."
Quinnab. Hashish (Arabic).
Quinnaq. Hashish (Arabic).
Quonnab. Hashish (Arabic).

_____ **R** _____

Rafi. Marihuana (Brazil).
Rahat Lakoum. Hashish confection (Turkey).
Rama. Marihuana (Central America).
Recetar. Sell marihuana (Costa Rica), literally "to prescribe." _See also_ Doctor, Medico, Pacientes.
Riamba. Marihuana (Brazil).
Rosa Maria. Marihuana (Mexico, Brazil).
Rubia, La. Marihuana (Colombia), literally "blonde one."
Rup. After flowers have been removed from marihuana plant to make ganja,* the rest of the plant is pulled out of ground and allowed to dry on a sheet in a closed room. Drying causes resin near top of plant to fall onto sheet. Resin is gathered and formed into a paste, which is very potent, called rup (India).

_____ **S** _____

Sabzi. Marihuana (South Africa).
Saffron. Hashish confection containing hashish, saffron oil, and fat. Mixture is molded into an orange-colored paste which is chewed (Egypt).
Sagrada. Marihuana (Mexico).
Sana. Marihuana (Sanskrit).
Sawi. Marihuana (India, Pakistan).
Semieniatka. Marihuana seed soup, prepared on Christmas Eve for spirits of dead family members who are believed to visit their relatives at this time (Lithuania, Poland).
Sentir se bonito. To begin to feel the effects of marihuana (Costa Rica), to feel a "buzz," literally "to feel pretty."
Sesame Sweetmeat. Hashish confection made with hashish, honey, and sesame seeds pressed into thin flat pieces.
Shakis. Marihuana (Nigeria).
Shesha. Hashish (Israel).
Shivbotty. Marihuana (India), literally "Shiva's plant."
Shora. Marihuana (Mexico).
Sibsa. Pipe for smoking hashish (Morocco).
Siddhi. Marihuana (India), literally "occult power."
Snuff. Marihuana (Nigeria).

Sonadora. Marihuana (Mexico).
Subjee. Marihuana (India).
Suknidhan. Marihuana (India).
Suma. Marihuana (Central Africa).
Suruma. Hashish (Mozambique).

T

Taco. Tobacco cigarette whose end is removed and filled with marihuana (Costa Rica), literally "wooden peg."
Tafe. Marihuana (Nigeria).
Tahgalm. Particles left over after powder is removed to make rup* (India).
Taju. Marihuana (Nigeria).
Takrouri. Hashish (Tunisia).
Tenebrosa. Marihuana smoker (Costa Rica), literally "gloomy one."
Teriaki. *See* Chatsraky.
Thandai. Marihuana (India).
Tiamba. Marihuana (Brazil).
Tieso. Intoxicated on marihuana (Costa Rica), literally "stiff."
Tiquira. Marihuana (Brazil).
Tirsa. Marihuana (Mexico).
Tocolo. Marihuana cigarette butt (Costa Rica).
Tosca. Marihuana (Central America).
Tostado. Chronic marihuana user (Costa Rica), literally "toasted."
Turba. Flat cake of hashish, weighing about one-half to two kilograms (Egypt).
Turkish Delight. *See* Malban.

U

Umburu. Marihuana (Brazil).
Uter. Hashish (Kashmir).

V

Vamos a prenderla. Smoke marihuana (Costa Rica), literally "let's set it on fire."
Verde. Marihuana (Costa Rica), literally "green."
Verdolaga. Marihuana (Mexico).
Vijaya. Marihuana (India), literally "victorious."
Vongony. Marihuana (Madagascar).

W

Wee Wee. Marihuana (Nigeria).

Y

Ya se llego. Initial effects of marihuana (Costa Rica), literally "it has come."
Yamba. Marihuana (Senegal).
Yerba. Marihuana (Costa Rica), literally "herb."

Z

Zamal. Marihuana (Madagascar, Réunion).
Zol. Marihuana cigarette (South Africa).
Zol rooker. Marihuana smoker (South Africa).

BIBLIOGRAPHY

Algren, N. *The Man with the Golden Arm.* New York: Doubleday & Co., 1949.

Anonymous. "A Hashish House in New York." *Harper's New Monthly Magazine* 67 (1883):944-49.

Anonymous. "The Menace of Marihuana." *International Medical Digest* 77 (1937): 183-87.

Anslinger, H. J. "Marihuana: Assassin of Youth." *American Magazine* 124 (1937): 18-19, 150-53.

———, and Oursler, W. *The Murderers.* New York: Avon, 1961.

Becker, H. S. *The Outsiders.* New York: Free Press, 1963.

Berger, M. "Tea for a Viper." *New Yorker*, March 12, 1938, pp. 47-50.

Berrey, L. V., and Van den Bark, M. *The American Thesaurus of Slang: A Complete Reference Book of Colloquial Speech.* New York: Thomas Y. Crowell, 1942.

Bevan, R. "Dope." *Everybody's*, June 12, 1954, pp. 11-13.

Black, W. *Dope, The Story of the Living Dead.* New York: Star Co., 1928.

Bloomquist, E. R. *Marihuana.* Beverly Hills, California: Glencoe Press, 1968.

Bouquet, J. "Cannabis." *Bulletin on Narcotics* 2 (1951):14-30.

Braddy, H. "Narcotic Argot Along the Mexican Border." *American Speech* 30 (1955):84-90.

———. "The Anonymous Verses of a Narcotic Addict." *Southern Folklore Quarterly*, September 1958, pp. 130-38.

Brennan, M. *Drugs*. San Antonio, Texas: Naylor Co., 1970.

Brown, C. *Manchild in the Promised Land*. 1965 rpt. New York: Macmillan, 1969.

Brown, J. D., ed. *The Hippies*. New York: Time, 1967.

Burley, D. *Dan Burley's Original Handbook of Harlem Jive*. Privately published, 1944.

Burroughs, W. S. *Junkie*. New York: Ace Books, 1953.

———. *Naked Lunch*. New York: Grove Press, 1959.

Calloway, C. *His Hi De Highness of Ho De Ho*. New York: Mills, 1935.

Carey, J. T. *The College Drug Scene*. Englewood Cliffs, New Jersey: Prentice Hall, 1968.

Carter, W. E., ed. *Cannabis in Costa Rica*. Philadelphia, Pennsylvania: Institute for Study of Human Issues, 1980.

Cavan, S. *Hippies of the Haight*. New York: New American Library, 1972.

Chandler, R. *Farewell, My Lovely*. New York: Pocket Books, 1943.

———. *The Little Sister*. 1949 rpt. New York: Ballantine Books, 1973.

———. *Playback*. 1958 rpt. New York: Ballantine Books, 1980.

Chaplin, M. *I Couldn't Smoke the Grass on My Father's Lawn*. New York: Ballantine Books, 1967.

Charen, S. and Perelman, L. "Personality studies of marihuana addicts." *American Journal of Psychiatry* 102 (1946):674-82.

Cherniak, L. *The Great Book of Hashish*. Berkeley, California: And-Or Press, 1979.

Chiardi, J. "Epitaph for the dead beats." *Saturday Review*, February 6, 1960, pp. 11-13, 42.

Claerbaut, D. *Black Jargon in White America*. New York: William B. Erdman, 1972.

Cooper, C. L. *The Scene*. New York: Crown Publishers, 1960.

Cooper, C. R. *Here's to Crime*. Boston, Massachusetts: Little, Brown, and Co., 1937.

Corley, E. *Acapulco Gold*. New York: Warner Books, 1974.

Coyote Man. *Get the Buzz On*. Berkeley, California: Brother William Press, 1972.

Cromwell, P. F. "Slang usage in the addict subculture." *Journal of Drug Issues* 1 (1970):75-78.

Danforth, H. R., and Horan, J. D. *Big City Crimes*. 1957 rpt. New York: Permabooks, 1960.

Dawtry, F. *Social Problems of Drug Abuse*. Woburn, Massachusetts: Butterworth, 1968.

de Farias, R. C. "Use of Maconha (*Cannabis Sativa 1*) in Brazil." *Bulletin on Narcotics* 7 (1955):5-19.

DeLeeuw, H. *Flower of Joy*. New York: Lee Furman, 1939.

De Lenoir, C. *The Hundredth Man*. New York: Claude Kendall, 1934.

De Mexico, N. R. *Marijuana Girl*. New York: Universal Publishers Co., 1960.

Duke, Osborn. *Sideman*. New York: Criterion Books, 1958.

Ellson H. *Reefer Boy*. London: Neville Spearman, 1955.

———. *Rock*. New York: Ballantine Books, 1955.

Eschholz, P. A., and Rosa, A. F. "Slang at the University of Vermont." *Current Slang* 5 (1971):1-10.

Farina, R. *Been Down So Long It Looks Like Up to Me.* New York: Dell, 1968.

Farmer, J. S., and Henley, W. E. *Slang and Its Analogues.* New York: Arno Press, 1970.

Farnsworth, N. R. "Pharacognosy and Chemistry of 'Cannabis Sativa.' " *Journal of the American Pharmaceutical Association* 9 (1969):410-14.

Folb, E. A. *A Comparative Study of Urban Black Argot.* Los Angeles, California: University of California, 1972.

Fossier, A. E. "The Marihuana Menace." *New Orleans Medical and Surgical Journal* 44 (1931):247-52.

Gardner, F. F. "New Mexico State University Slang." *Current Slang* 4 (1970): 1-26.

Geller, A., and Boas, M. *The Drug Beat.* New York: Cowles Book Co., 1969.

Gladstone, T. H. *The Englishman in Kansas.* 1857 rpt. Lincoln: University of Nebraska, 1971.

Gold, R. S. *Jazz Lexicon.* Indianapolis, Indiana: Bobbs-Merrill Co., 1979.

Goldin, H. E., O'Leary, F., and Lipsius, B. *Dictionary of American Underworld Lingo.* New York: Twayne Publishers, 1950.

Goldman, A. *Grass Roots.* New York: Warner Books, 1980.

Goldstein, R. "The College Scene in the U.S.A." In G. Andrews and S. Vinkmoog (eds.), *Book of Grass.* New York: Grove Press, 1967, pp. 214-18.

Gomerly, S. *Drugs and the Canadian Scene.* Toronto: Burns and Macechern, 1970.

Goode, E., ed. *Marijuana.* Chicago, Illinois: Atherton, 1969.

———. *The Marijuana Smokers.* New York: Basic Books, 1970.

Gottschalk, L. A., and Cowdry, F. V. *The Language of the Narcotic Addict.* Paper presented at the U.S. Public Health Service Hospital, Fort Worth, Texas, 1948.

Gross, H. *The Flower People.* New York: Ballantine Books, 1968.

Hall, P. *Heads, You Lose.* New York: Hawthorn Books, 1971.

Harris, J. D. *The Junkie Priest.* 1964 rpt. New York: Pocket Books, 1965.

Hayes, M. H., and Bowery, L. E. "Marihuana." *Journal of Criminology* 23 (1933): 1086-97.

Heard, N. C. *Howard Street.* New York: Dial Press, 1968.

Himes, C. *For Love of Imabelle.* New York: Signet Books, 1965.

———. "Marihuana and a pistol." *Esquire,* March 1940, p. 28.

Holiday, B. *Lady Sings the Blues.* 1956 rpt. New York: Lancer Books, 1959.

Holmes, J. C. *The Horn.* 1953 rpt. New York: Random House, 1959.

Housley, L. B. *A Dictionary of Underground Slang.* Seattle, Washington: Columbia Publishing Co., 1939.

Hughes, H. M. *The Fantastic Lodge.* Boston: Houghton-Mifflin, 1961.

Hughes, L., and Bontemps, A. *The Book of Negro Folklore.* New York: Dodd, Mead, 1958.

Hunter, E. *Second Ending.* New York: Simon and Schuster, 1956.

Iceberg Slim. *Pimp, The Story of My Life.* Los Angeles, California: Holloway House Publishing Co., 1969.

Indian Hemp Drugs Commission Report. London: Government Printing Office, 1893-1894.

Irish, W. *Marihuana*. New York: Dell, 1941.

Isyurhash, M., and Rusoff, G. *The Gourmet Guide to Grass*. New York: Pinnacle Books, 1974.

Jamer, R. *Hippie Sex Communes*. Los Angeles: Impact Books, 1970.

Jones, M., and Chilton, J. *Louis*. Boston, Massachusetts: Little, Brown, and Co., 1971.

Kaplan, J. H. "Marijuana and Drug Abuse in Vietnam." *Annals of the New York Academy of Sciences* 191 (1970):261-69.

Kerouac, J. *On the Road*. 1955 rpt. New York: Penguin Books, 1980.

———. *The Subterraneans*. New York: Grove Press, 1958.

King, A. *Mine Enemy Grows Older*. New York: Signet Books, 1960.

La Guardia Committee on Marihuana. *The Marihuana Problem in the City of New York*. 1944 rpt. Metuchen, New Jersey: Scarecrow Reprint Corp., 1973.

Lait, J., and Mortimer, L. *Washington Confidential*. New York: Dell, 1951.

Landy, E. E. *The Underground Dictionary*. New York: Simon and Schuster, 1971.

Lannoy, W. C., and Masterson, E. "Teen-Age Hophead Jargon." *American Speech* (1952):23-31.

Laurie, P. *Drugs*. Middlesex, England: Penguin Books, 1971.

Le Dain Commission. *Cannabis*. Ottawa: Information Canada, 1972.

Lentini, J. R. *Vice and Narcotics Control*. Beverly Hills, California: Glencoe Press, 1977.

Lindesmith, A. R. *The Addict and the Law*. New York: Vintage Books, 1967.

Lipton, L. *The Holy Barbarians*. New York: Grove Press, 1959.

Longstreet, S. *The Real Jazz Old and New*. Baton Rouge, Louisiana: State University Press, 1956.

Lubin, S. *Hippies, Drugs, and Promiscuity*. New Rochelle, New York: Arlington House, 1972.

Mandell, G. *Flee the Angry Strangers*. New York: Bobbs-Merrill Co., 1952.

Manning, J. *Reefer Girl*. New York: Cameo Books, 1953.

Marcovitz, E., and Myers, H. J. "The Marihuana Addict in the Army." *War Medicine* 6 (1944):382-91.

Margolis, J. S., and Clorfene, R. *A Child's Garden of Grass*. 1969 rpt. New York: Pocket Books, 1970.

Marsten, R. *So Nude, So Dead*. New York: Fawcett, 1956.

Mathews, M. M. *A Dictionary of Americanisms*. Chicago: University of Chicago Press, 1951.

Maurer, D. M. "The Argot of the Underworld Narcotic Addict." *American Speech* 11 (1936):116-27; 179-92.

———, and Vogel, V. H. *Narcotic and Narcotics Addiction*. Springfield, Illinois: C. C. Thomas, 1954.

McCullers, C. *The Ballad of the Sad Café*. New York: Houghton-Mifflin Co., 1951.

Mezzrow, M., and Wolfe, B. *Really the Blues*. New York: Dell, 1946.

Monteleone, V. J. *Criminal Slang*. Boston, Massachusetts: Christopher Publishing House, 1949.

Murtagh, J. M., and Harris, S. *Who Live in Shadows*. New York: McGraw-Hill, 1959.

Newton, F. *The Jazz Scene.* London: MacGibbon and Kee, 1959.

Nicholas, T. *Rastafari.* Garden City, New York: Anchor, 1979.

Novak, W. *High Culture.* New York: Alfred A. Knopf, 1980.

Oursler, W., and Smith, L. D. *Hooked.* New York: Popular Library, 1952.

Partridge, E. *A Dictionary of the Underworld.* New York: Bonanza Books, 1961.

Pollock, A. J. *The Underworld Speaks.* San Francisco, California: Prevent Crime Bureau, 1935.

Polsky, N. *Hustlers, Beats and Others.* New York: Doubleday, 1967. rpt. 1969.

Pritchie, N. *The Savage Kick.* New York: Fawcett, 1962.

Rechy, J. *City of Night.* New York: Grove Press, 1963.

Rettig, R. P., Torres, M., and Garrett, G. R. *Manny, A Criminal Addict's Story.* Boston, Massachusetts: Houghton-Mifflin, 1977.

Ric. "I Turned on 200 Fellow Students at the University of Michigan." *Esquire* 101 (1937):190-93.

Rosevear, J. *Pot.* New York: Lancer, 1967.

Rowell, E. A. *Adventures of David Dare.* Hinsdale, Illinois: Privately published, 1938.

Russell, R. *The Sound.* New York: E. P. Dutton, 1961.

Sanders, E. *Shards of God.* New York: Grove Press, 1970.

Saxon, L., Dreyer, E., and Tallant, R. *Gumbo Ya Ya.* Boston, Massachusetts: Houghton-Mifflin, 1945.

Schiano, A. *Solo.* New York: Warner Books, 1974.

Schmidt, J. E. *Narcotics Lingo and Lore.* Springfield, Illinois: C. C. Thomas, 1959.

Schwartz, A. *The Blowtop.* New York: Dial Press, 1948.

Selby, H. *Last Exit to Brooklyn.* New York: Grove Press, 1957.

Shorris, E. *Ofay.* New York: Dell, 1967.

Silver, G., and Aldrich, M. *Dope Chronicles.* New York: Harper and Row, 1979.

Simmons, J. L., ed. *Marihuana.* North Hollywood, California: Brandon House, 1967.

Siragusa, C. *The Trail of the Poppy.* Englewood Cliffs, New Jersey: Prentice-Hall, 1966.

Smith, D. E., and Gray, G. R. *It's So Good, Don't Even Try It Once.* Englewood Cliffs, New Jersey: Prentice-Hall, 1972.

Smith, R. F. Report of Investigation in the State of Texas, Particularly along the Mexican Border, of the Traffic in, and Consumption of the Drug Generally Known as 'Indian Hemp' or *Cannabis Indica.* United States Department of Agriculture, April 13, 1917.

Smith, W. *The Little Tigress.* 1923 rpt. Freeport, New York: Books for Libraries Press, 1971.

Smith, W. G. *Anger at Innocence.* 1950 rpt. Chatham, New Jersey: Chatham Bookseller, 1973.

Sorfleet, P. "Dealing Hashish." *Canadian Journal of Criminology* 18 (1976):123-51.

Southern, T. "Red Dirt Marihuana." In D. Solomon (ed.), *Marihuana Papers.* New York: Signet, 1967.

Spencer, R. R. "Marijuana." *Health Officer* 1 (1936):299-305.

Spitzmiller, O. "The Head Community as Deviant Subculture." *Folklore Annual of the University Folklore Association, University of Texas* 1 (1969):1-10.

St. Johns, A. R. "Walking on Air." *Hearst's International Cosmopolitan* 104 (1938): 36-39, 103-10.

Stanley, E. "Marihuana as a Developer of Criminals." *American Journal of Police Science* 2 (1931):252-61.

Sullivan, M. *My Double Life.* New York: Farrar and Rinehart, 1938.

Sutter, A. G. "The World of the Righteous Dope Fiend." *Issues in Criminology* 2 (1966):177-222.

Thomas, P. *Down These Mean Streets.* New York: Signet Books, 1967.

Thorpe, R. *Hooked.* New York: Paperback Library, 1956.

Trocchi, A. *Cain's Book.* 1960 rpt. New York: Grove Press, 1961.

Trujillo, E. *I Love You, I Hate You.* New York: Levy, 1955.

University of California, *Folklore Archives.* "Narcotics."

Wallop, D. *Night Light.* New York: William Norton, 1953.

Walton, R. P. *Marihuana.* Philadelphia, Pennsylvania: J. P. Lippincott, 1958.

Weber, C. M. "Mary Warner." *Health Digest* 3 (1936):77-80.

Wentworth, H., and Flexner, S. B. *Dictionary of American Slang.* New York: Thomas Y. Crowell, 1975.

Westin, A. and Shaffer, S. *Heroes and Heroin.* New York: Pocket Books, 1972.

White, W. "Wayne University Slang." *American Speech* 30 (1955):301-5.

Williams, J. B., ed. *Narcotics and Hallucinogens.* Beverly Hills, California: Glencoe Press, 1969.

Wilson, E. "Crazy Dreamers." *Collier's* 123 (1949):27.

Winick, C. "Marihuana Use by Young People." In E. Harms (ed.), *Drug Addiction in Youth.* Oxford: Pergamon Press, 1965, pp. 19-35.

Witmore, S. *Solo.* New York: Harcourt Brace, 1955.

Wolf, W. "Uncle Sam Fights a New Drug Menace . . . Marihuana." *Popular Science Monthly* 128 (1936):14-15, 119-20.

Wolfe, B. H. *Hippies.* St. Louis: New Critics Press, 1968.

Woodley, R. *Dealer.* New York: Holt, Rinehart, and Winston, 1971.

Wylie, P. *Finnley Wren.* New York: Rinehart, 1934.

Yawger, N. S. "Marihuana, Our New Addiction." *American Journal of Medical Science* 195 (1938):351-57.

INDEX

About the Author

ERNEST L. ABEL is a research scientist at the Research Institute on Alcoholism, and a specialist in behavioral teratology. He is the author of several books, including *Handwriting on the Wall: Toward a Sociology and Psychology of Graffiti* (Greenwood Press, 1977) and *A Comprehensive Guide to the Cannabis Literature* (Greenwood Press, 1979).